A Practical Guide to Clinical Application of OCT in Ophthalmology

Edited by Michele Lanza

Published in London, United Kingdom

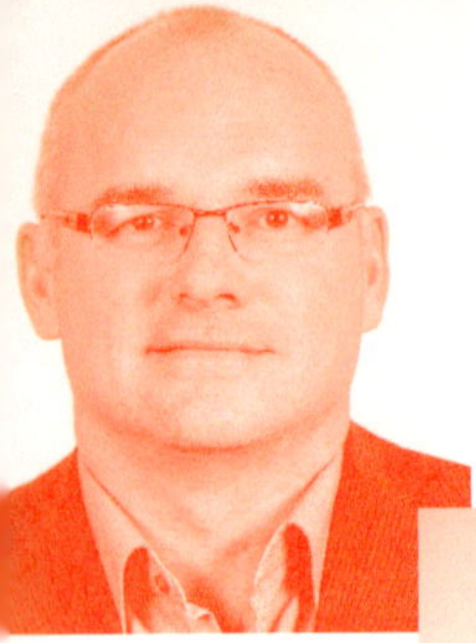
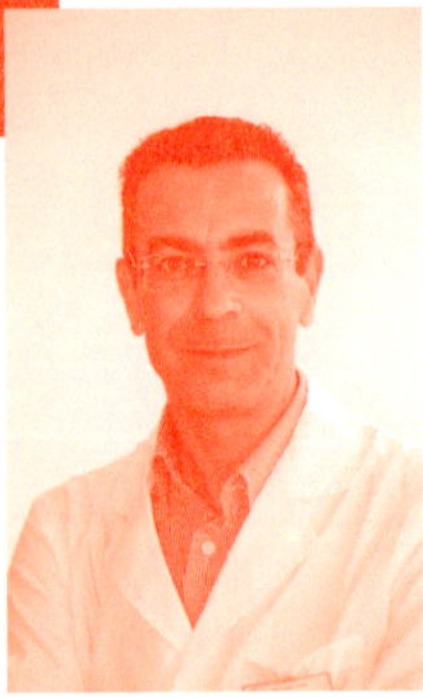
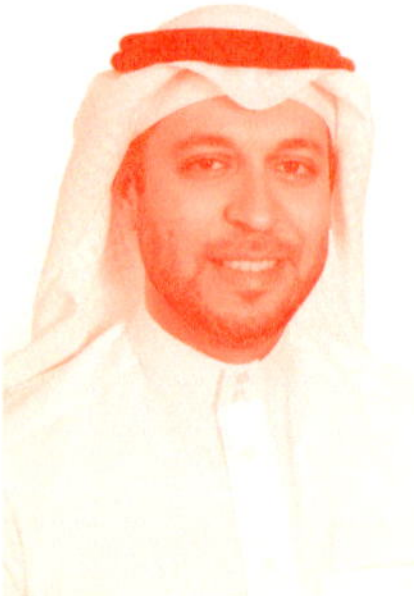
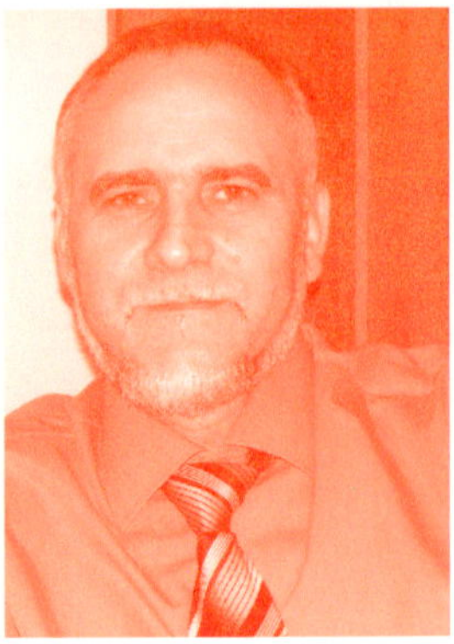
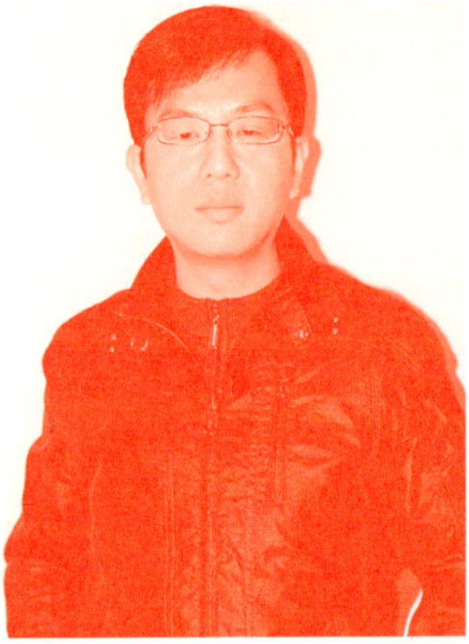
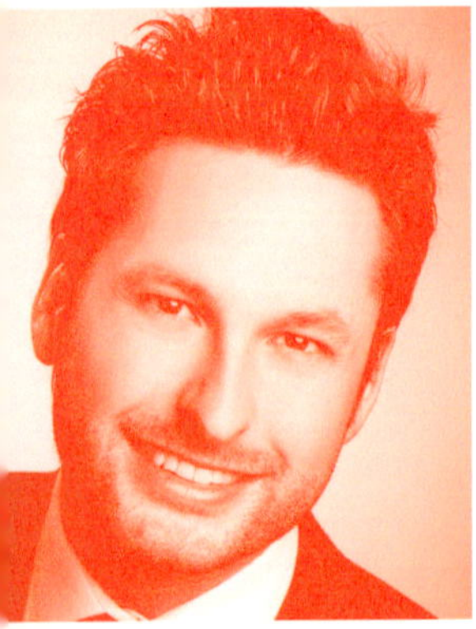
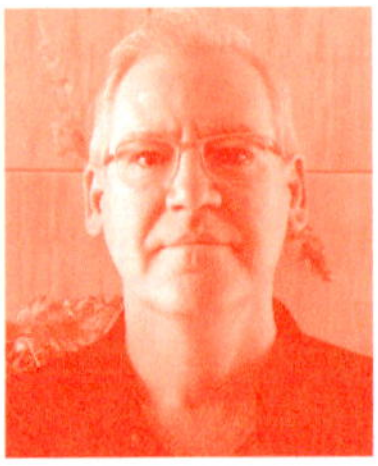

IntechOpen

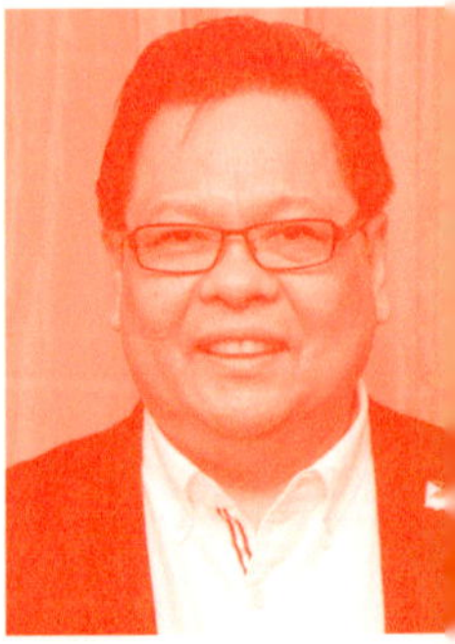
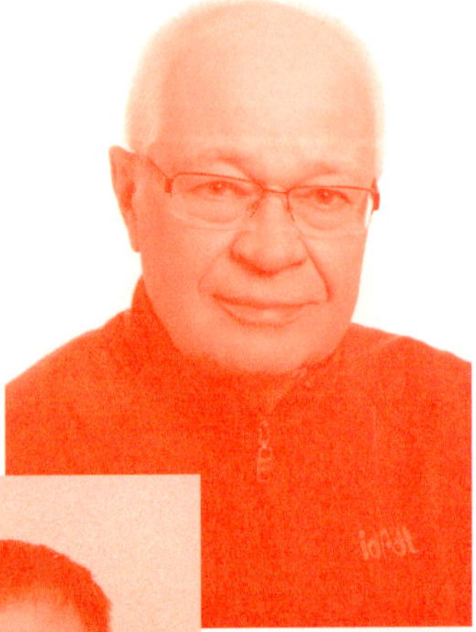
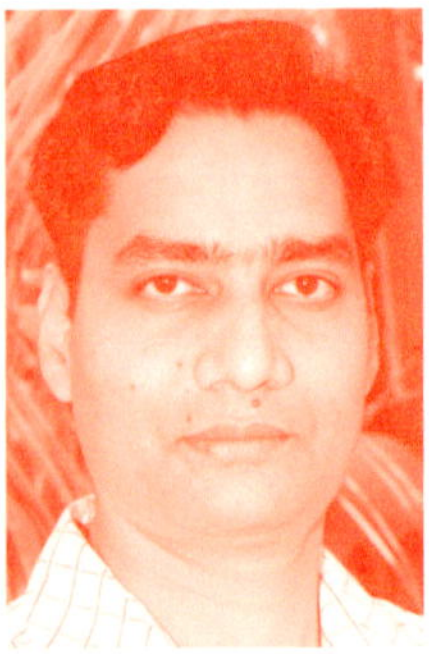
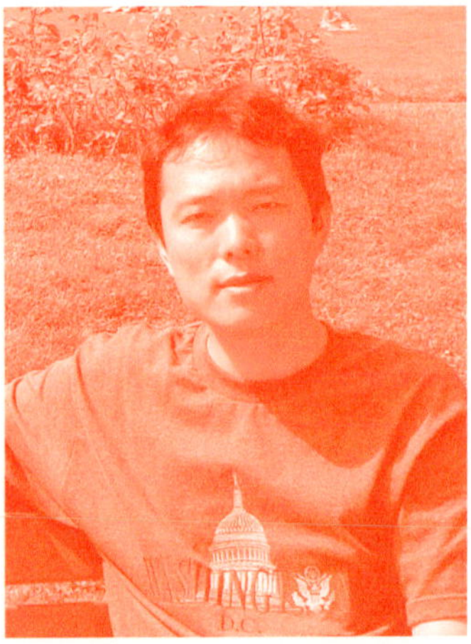
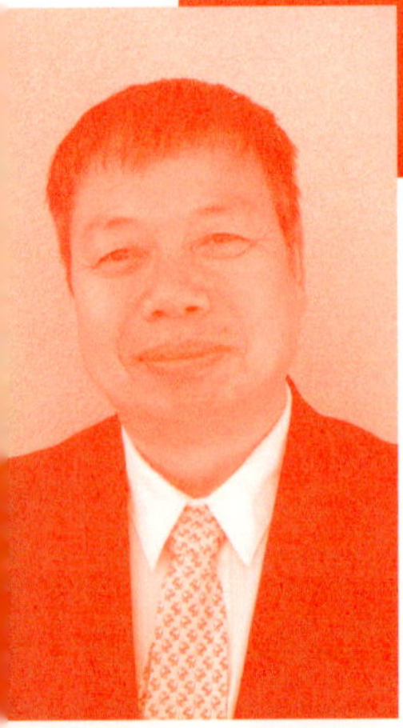
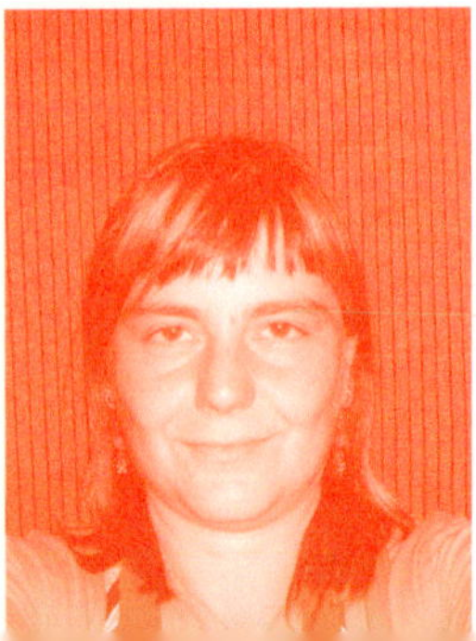

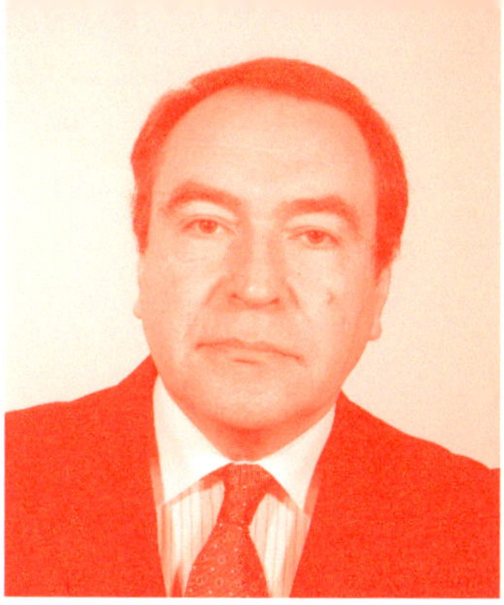
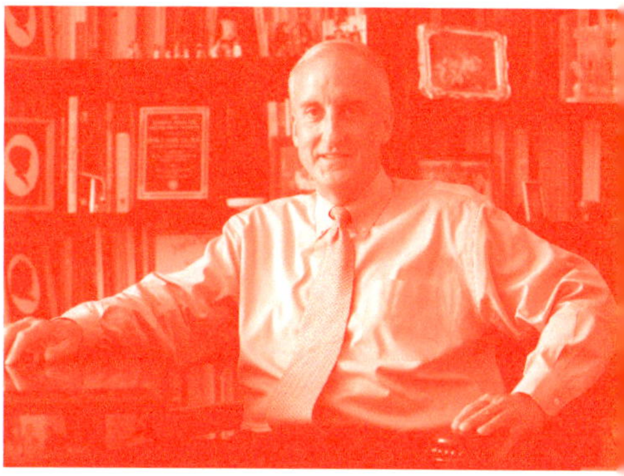
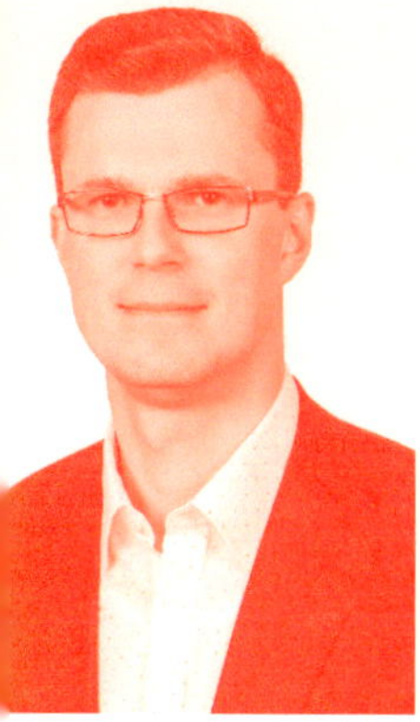
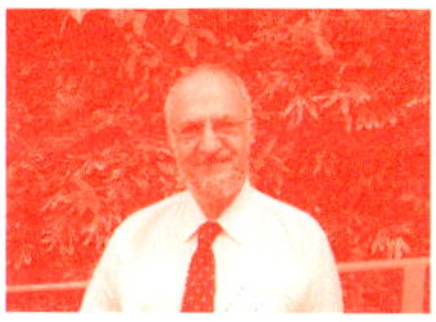
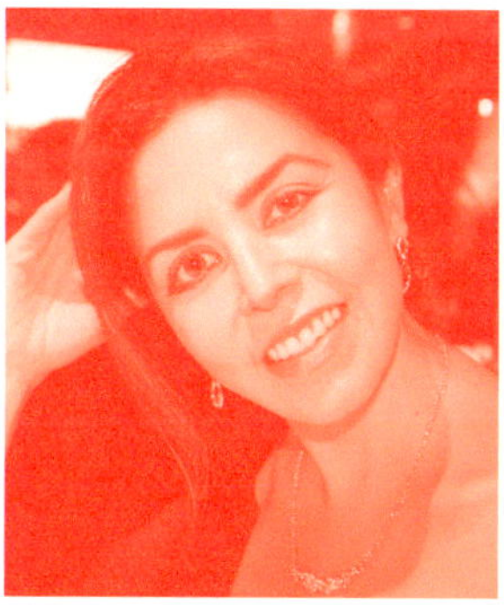

Supporting open minds since 2005

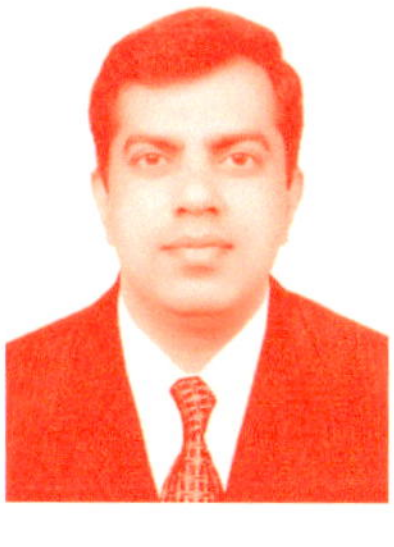
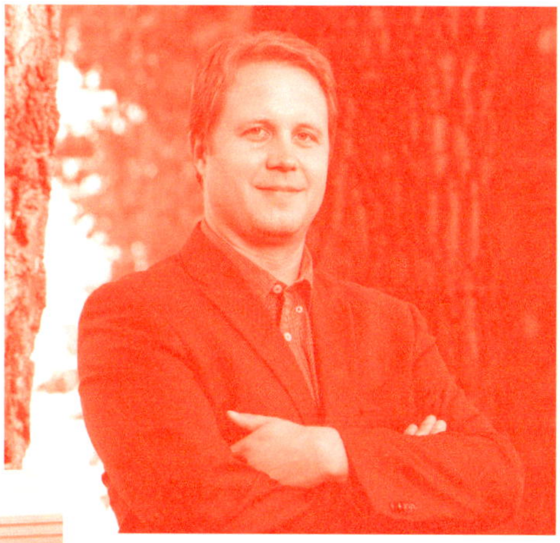
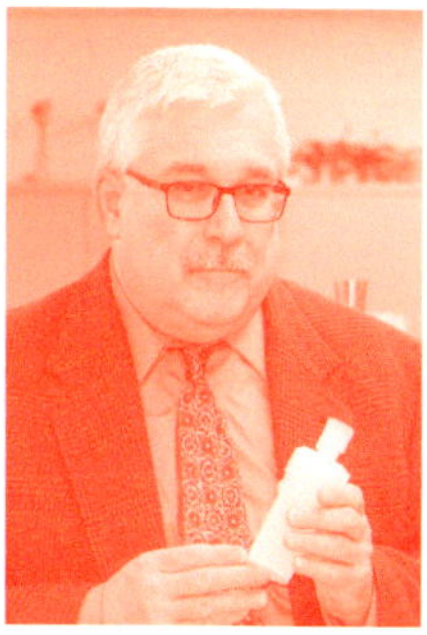
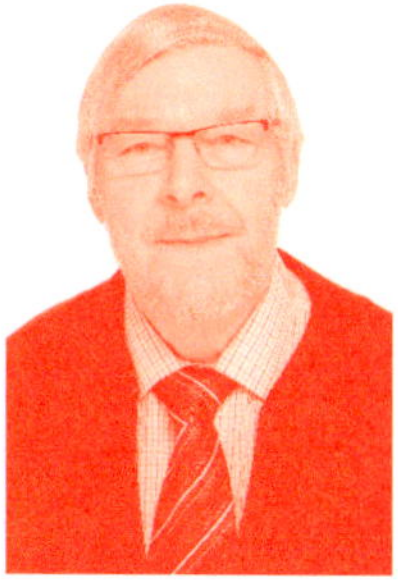
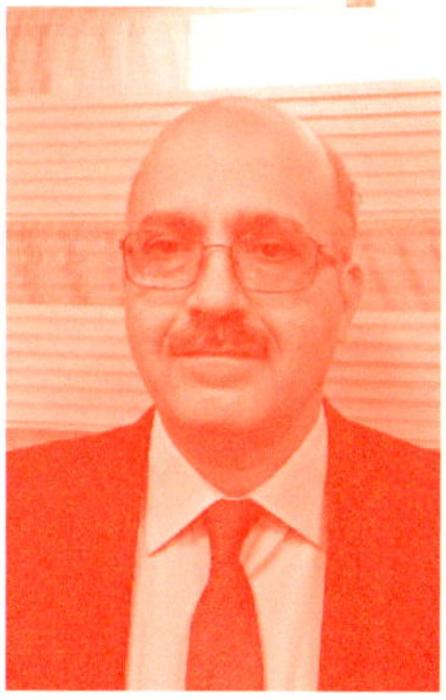
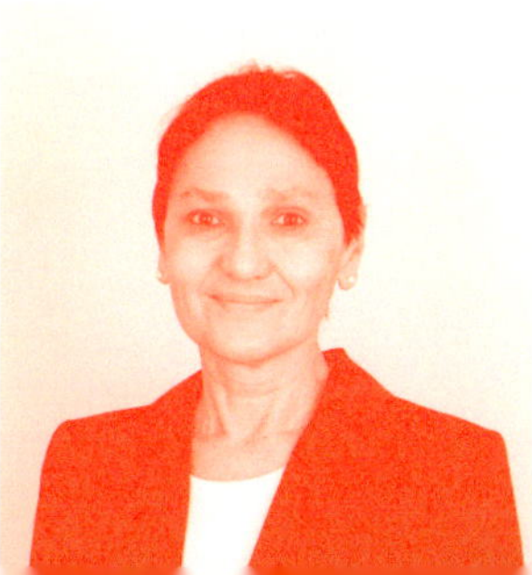
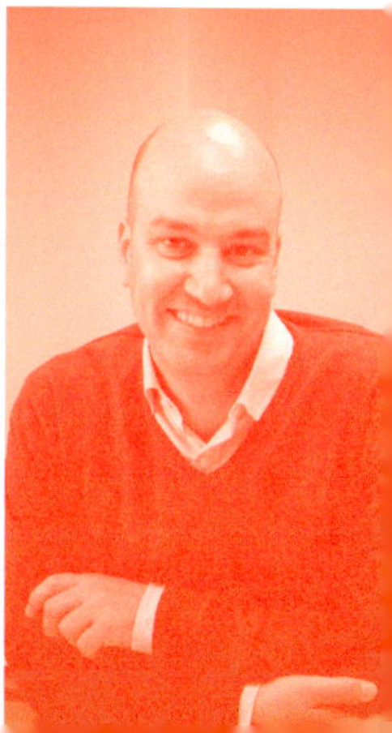

A Practical Guide to Clinical Application of OCT in Ophthalmology
http://dx.doi.org/10.5772/intechopen.77676
Edited by Michele Lanza

Contributors
Baswati Sahoo, Julie Pegu, Magdy Moussa, Mahmoud Leila, Naresh Kumar Yadav, Ramesh Venkatesh, Bharathi Bavaharan, Raffaele Piscopo, Mario Bifani, Michele Lanza, Luigi Mele, Constanza Caramello, María Ángeles Del Buey, Paula Casas, Enrique Mínguez, Sara Marco, Francisco J. Ascaso, Reza Ghaffari, Hassan Hashemi, Soheila Asgari, Javier Lara Medina, Olivia Esteban Floria, Carmen Ispa Callén, Javier Mateo, Isabel Bartolomé, Jane Cook, Vatookarn Roongpoovapatr, Taher Eleiwa, Sonia Yoo, Mohamed Abou Shousha

First published in London, United Kingdom, 2019 by IntechOpen
IntechOpen is the global imprint of INTECHOPEN LIMITED, registered in England and Wales, registration number: 11086078, The Shard, 25th floor, 32 London Bridge Street
London, SE19SG – United Kingdom
Printed in Croatia

British Library Cataloguing-in-Publication Data
A catalogue record for this book is available from the British Library

Additional hard and PDF copies can be obtained from orders@intechopen.com

A Practical Guide to Clinical Application of OCT in Ophthalmology
Edited by Michele Lanza
p. cm.
Print ISBN 978-1-78984-015-5
Online ISBN 978-1-78984-016-2
eBook (PDF) ISBN 978-1-83962-220-5

For EU product safety concerns:
IN TECH d.o.o., Prolaz Marije Krucifikse Kozulić 3, 51000 Rijeka, Croatia, info@intechopen.com or visit our website at intechopen.com.

Meet the editor

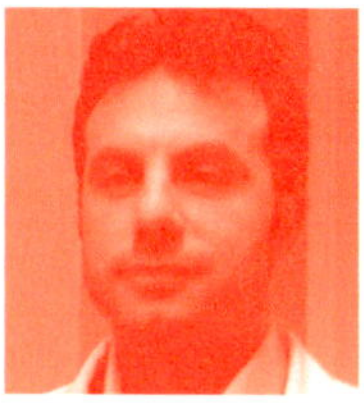

Michele Lanza, PhD, MD, graduated in medicine (2001) and completed his residency program in ophthalmology (2005) at Seconda Università di Napoli, Italy. He also obtained a PhD degree in Biomechanical Engineering at Biomedical Engineering Silesian University of Technology, Zabrze, Poland (2018). Currently, he is an assistant professor at Università della Campania Luigi Vanvitelli, Napoli, Italy. He has been a principal investigator and participant in research projects granted by his own university and by other national agencies, a teacher in the school of medicine, and organized courses at national and international conferences. He obtained the Achievement Award of the American Academy of Ophthalmology (2017). He is the author of more than 160 papers in national and international conferences, 60 papers in impact factor journals, and four chapters in Italian books. His fields of interest are refractive surgery, glaucoma, cataract surgery, and ocular complication of neurological diseases.

Contents

Preface

This book aims to provide readers with new applications of optical coherence tomography (OCT) during clinical practice. The first section will focus on diseases affecting the cornea and conjunctiva: OCT is a posterior segment, traditionally used diagnostic device but is now very useful and interesting in evaluating the whole eyeball. Physicians will be able to recognize the most significant signs of described diseases to better handle them, making both earlier diagnosis and appropriate therapies possible. OCT defines new standards to recognize and standardize inflammation marks and this could be very useful for physicians facing diseases that could provide very aspecific signs and symptoms. In particular, diseases affecting the conjunctiva have not previously been studied with OCT, so this could be an exciting new prospect for OCT and is also focused on in this section.

The second section shows the application of OCT in macular diseases and new standards and definitions that are possible to obtain the latest version of this device. These improvements in the definition and precision of OCT scans are extremely useful to obtain help for early recognition of macular diseases and to apply proper treatments. New therapies purposed for macular diseases appear to be very promising but timing is a very crucial factor to obtain satisfactory results. Glaucoma patients are now undergoing OCT to recognize early defects of the disease before visual field defects appear. Moreover, to study retinal nerve fiber layers in these patients is helpful especially for those who have very deep visual impairment or other problems that do not allow them to perform a reliable visual field test. Chapters related to this topic will guide readers through the usefulness of OCT in evaluating glaucoma patients.

At the end of the book readers will have the chance to evaluate the usefulness of OCT in every ocular field and will have an idea of the new frontiers that are going to be overcome. I would like to thank all the authors and coauthors who worked hard in providing very high-quality chapters, and the editorial staff who made this book possible.

Michele Lanza, MD, PhD
Università degli Studi della Campania "Luigi Vanvitelli",
Italy

Section 1

OCT in Corneal and External Disease

Chapter 1

Corneal Microlayer Optical Tomography Review

Vatookarn Roongpoovapatr, Jane C. Cook, Taher K. Eleiwa, Sonia H. Yoo and Mohamed Abou Shousha

Abstract

Anterior segment ultra-high resolution OCT (UHR-OCT) uses a resolution of 1–4 μm to provide non-invasive imaging of the tear film and cornea. This new high definition imaging technology increases our understanding of normal structure and pathological changes in the cornea, and resolution has continued to improve over time. UHR-OCT is useful in the treatment of disease such as dry eye, subclinical keratoconus, keratoconus, and ocular surface pathology. It also aids clinicians in fitting contact lenses and screening tissue for corneal transplantation. In this review, we summarize applications of imaging the normal and pathologic ocular surface and cornea. Novel developments, such as the new-generation micro-OCT, Anterior segment OCT angiography and artificial intelligence have the potential to continue to increase our knowledge.

Keywords: optical coherence tomography, optical biopsy, corneal microlayer, graft rejection, corneal imaging

1. Introduction

Speed and image quality of Optical Coherence Tomography (OCT) technology have made great strides over the past few decades [1–3]. OCT has long been a critical part of imaging the posterior segment, but is now starting to become more helpful for the anterior segment as well [3].

As anterior segment OCT has evolved, the precision of axial resolution has increased, from 15 to 20 μm resolution of time domain (TD-OCT) to 4–7 μm of spectral domain (SD-OCT) and Fourier-domain OCT (FD-OCT) and 1–4 μm of Ultra- high resolution OCT (UHR-OCT) [4, 5]. Speed has improved and UHR-OCT allows for real-time imaging and minimizes motion artifacts compared with older models [6–8]. Scan width of UHR-OCT has also improved to the current 5–12 mm [2–9].

This high definition imaging shows the *in vivo* pathological changes in microlayers of the cornea. Many publications have described the utility of UHR-OCT in clinical diagnosis and management of corneal disease [2, 10–13]. In the following review, we summarize the clinical applications of imaging the ocular surface and cornea based on anatomical structure and will focus on UHR-OCT.

IntechOpen

2. Ultra-high resolution OCT

2.1 Technical aspects

Optical coherence tomography (OCT) is a non-contact image acquisition technology first developed by Huang et al. [14]. It produces an 'optical biopsy': detailed cross-sectional images of biological tissue [14]. Signal acquisition and processing methods determine image speed and resolution [15]. As resolution and tissue penetrance have improved, clinical applications continue to evolve [16].

The time-domain OCT (TD-OCT) was the first available anterior segment OCT, with the prototypes Visante and SL-OCT (Heidelberg Engineering, Heidelberg, Germany). Both acquired 2000 A-scans per second and had a resolution of 10–18 μm. These earlier models could scan the entire anterior segment, but were slow with poor resolution [1, 2]. Resolution improved to 5 μm with the SD-OCT, but scan width was limited at 3–6 mm. Available SD-OCTs included the Cirrus (Carl Zeiss Meditec, Inc.), Spectralis (Heidelberg Engineering, Dossenheim, Germany), RTVue (Optovue, Meridianville, AL), 3D OCT (Topcon Medical Systems, Oakland, NJ), and Bioptigen SD-OCT (Bioptigen Inc., Research Triangle Park, NC) [1, 2]. Swept-source (SS) Fourier-domain (FD) OCT was available in 2008 and the prototype was Casia SS OCT (Tomey, Nagoya, Japan). This SS-OCT had a scan width of 16 mm, depth of 6 mm and A-scan rate of 30,000 per second which then allowed for three-dimensional scanning of the entire anterior segment [1].

The first use of UHR-OCT was reported by Drexler et al. in 2001 with 2–3 resolution imaging of Bowman's membrane [17]. Current axial resolution of the UHR-OCT is 1–4 μm with a scan width of 5–12 mm [9, 10, 18]. OCT resolution was improved with a light source with a broad bandwidth greater than 100 nm and a specifically designed spectrometer which detected fringes collected from both reference and sample arms [2]. These changes allowed for *in vivo* imaging of individual corneal layers (microlayer), the tear film, tear meniscus and contact lens interfaces [9, 18, 19].

Most published data using UHR-OCT was acquired from custom-built machines, and availability. The Bioptigen Envisu (Bioptigen Inc., Research Triangle Park, NC, USA) and the SOCT Copernicus HR (Optopol Technologies SA, Zawiercie, Poland) are current commercially available models of UHR-OCT.

2.2 Corneal anatomy

The cornea is the transparent structure which, along with the tear film, provides about two-thirds of the refractive power of the eye [20]. The central cornea on average is 551–565 μm thick and the peripheral cornea ranges from 612 to 640 μm thick [21]. The cornea receives its nutrients mainly from the aqueous humor, as it is an avascular structure. Cellular components of the cornea include epithelial cells, keratocytes, and endothelial cells. Acellular components of the cornea form a matrix of collagen and glycosaminoglycans. Corneal transparency is based on uniformity of collagen fibril diameter and packing [22].

2.3 Healthy cornea parameters

UHR-OCT of the healthy cornea is important in order to recognize changes in disease states (**Figure 1**). UHR-OCT parameters of the normal tear film were first reported by Werkmeister et al. [10]. The group reported an average central tear

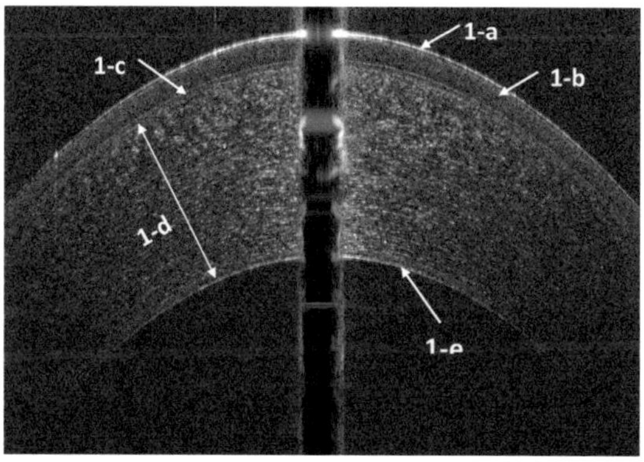

Figure 1.
A prototypical cross-sectional UHR-OCT image of a healthy human cornea. Epithelium (1b), Bowman's layer (1c), stroma (1d), and endothelium/ Descemet membrane complex (1e) can be distinguished. The topmost highly reflective layer in the tomogram represents the pre-corneal tear film (1-a).

film thickness of 4.79 μm [23]. Other reported central tear film thicknesses include 3.4 μm [24], 5.1 μm [25] and a range of 3–8 μm [26]. The central cornea measured 585 μm, with epithelial thicknesses of 55 [10] and 55.8 μm [25].

Data from a SD-OCT with 3.9 μm axial resolution showed that central corneal epithelium thickness is not statistically significant between subjects less than or greater than 40 years old (48.3 and 48.8 μm, respectively) [27]. This conclusion was supported by previous studies which showed no alteration in epithelial cell density with age [28]. Epithelial thickness varied over the vertical and horizontal meridians from 42.9 to 55.2 μm and 58.6 to 59.3 μm, respectively [29].

Bowman's layer has been reported as 18 [10] and 18.7 μm [25] thick with an uneven thickness distribution over the horizontal meridian of the cornea [25]. The central and midperiphery, nasal, temporal Bowman's layer thickness was 17.7, 20.0 and 19.8 μm, respectively [25]. Thickness gradually increases from temporal to nasal and from inferior to superior [25].

The Endothelium/Descemet membrane complex (En/DM) is made of Descemet membrane (DM), endothelium, and retro-corneal membranes. These layers are typically indistinguishable so the thickness measured from UHR-OCT is different from that from pathology [30]. DM in healthy young subjects is seen with UHR-OCT as a single, opaque, smooth line. The same structure is a band of two smooth opaque lines surrounding a translucent space in normal elderly subjects [9]. Bizheva et al. reported UHR-OCT data from healthy subjects, and revealed the average thickness was 6.6 for pre-Descemet's layer, 10.4 μm for Descemet's membrane and 4.8 μm for endothelium [31]. Another group published an average central Descemet's membrane thicknesses of 10 and 16 μm in the young and elderly healthy groups, respectively [9].

2.4 Applications of UHR-OCT for corneal microlayers

Corneal imaging has been significantly improved by the improvements in speed and resolution in the current UHR-OCT. The high axial resolution of UHR-OCT systems allows precise delineation of the corneal microlayers. There are a wide variety of clinical applications of UHR-OCT for the diagnosis and management of corneal disease [12, 13, 16, 17]. In this review, we summarize the clinical applications of imaging the ocular surface and cornea based on microlayers of the cornea.

3. Corneal pathology within the tear film

3.1 Dry eye and tear evaluation

OCT assessment of the tear meniscus has been extensively studied during the last 10 years [32]. The pathophysiology of dry eye disease is characterized by instability of the pre-corneal tear film along with increased osmolarity and ocular surface inflammation and damage [33]. Anterior segment OCT imaging in patients with dry eye disease is clinically useful as it can help directly image the tear film, Meibomian glands and conjunctival folds.

Tear film imaging is inherently limited by the fact that the tear film constantly changes with blinking [1, 23, 24, 34, 35]. OCT meniscometry solves this problem by continuously measuring the tear film, using a tear meniscus to represent the total volume. This method of acquiring images is objective, non-invasive and rapid [32, 34]. However, data analysis is complex, operator-dependent and time-consuming [36]. Tear meniscus height, curvature, and cross-sectional area are widely used in clinical practice and demonstrate good diagnostic performance and correlations with other tests [32, 34].

Cui et al. reported the first visualization of the pre-corneal tear film in dry eye patients with UHR-OCT [12]. The patients were asked to blink normally and then delay each blink as long as possible. The average pre-corneal tear film significantly increased from 4.4 μm during normal blinking to 6.6 μm during delayed blinking. The lipid layer of the tear film can be directly visualized using a contrast mechanism based on sample OCT reflectance, and measures 40–80 nm [37]. The tear film also increases on UHR-OCT after the use of artificial tears and punctal occlusion [38–41].

3.2 Contact lens fitting

UHR-OCT can perform a dynamic evaluation of contact lens movement with blinking and shifting gaze [42]. Soft contact lenses usually overlap 2 mm on the bulbar conjunctiva, but can displace further and overlap 4 to 5 mm onto the bulbar conjunctiva during blinking [43]. UHR-OCT can image the location of the edge of the lens and the tear film underneath the periphery of the lens. This data can help us to understand the normal physiology of the tear film and the dry eye associated with contact lens wear.

The tear film allows contact lens wearers to maintain vision and comfort and health [44]. Lens adherence and ocular surface staining can result from a decreased tear film [43]. Both pre-lens and post-lens tear film contribute to contact lens-associated dry eye [44]. Chen et al. imaged the tear film of 22 subjects before and after contact lens wear with a 15 mm scan width and 3 μm resolution UHR-OCT. Data showed that the pre-lens tear film increased after the instillation of artificial tears, whereas the post-lens tear film remained the same [18]. Cui et al. used UHR-OCT to study soft contact lens conjunctival overlap and the post-lens tear film. They found that increased conjunctival overlap was associated with reduced post-lens tear film underneath the peripheral region of soft contact lens during lens daily wear. Contact lenses with rounded edges also had more conjunctival overlap than the lenses with angled edges [43].

4. Corneal epithelial pathology

4.1 Dry eye

Artificial tears eye drops use increased central corneal epithelial and mid-peripheral corneal thickness in dry eye patients. Epithelial thickness can be a useful measurement when evaluating treatment response in dry eye patients, but the pattern of epithelial changes in this disease remains inconclusive [45]. The epithelium has been reported to be thinner [46–47], the same [48], and thicker [49] in dry eye patients in several conflicting studies. Central epithelial thickness in female dry eye patients was thicker than that of normal control patients by 6.5 and 6.2 μm, respectively [49]. Further cell morphology studies may be warranted to differentiate the possible explanations of increased epithelial thickness associated with dry eye. Epithelial hypertrophy or hyperplasia, edema, or increased number of cellular layers may be contributing [49]. Abou Shousha et al. demonstrated that dry eye patients had increased corneal epithelial irregularity compared to controls, quantified by corneal epithelial thickness profile variance and range. Both parameters were significantly correlated with questionnaire scores and improved after dry eye treatment [50].

4.2 Subclinical keratoconus

Xu et al. reported UHR-OCT epithelial vertical thickness profiles in the diagnosis of subclinical keratoconus. Data showed statistically significant thinning of the central corneal epithelium; 53.48 μm in normal eyes and 51.92 μm in those with subclinical keratoconus. There was no significant inferior epithelial thinning in subclinical keratoconus; 54.94 μm in normal eyes and 54.85 μm in eyes with subclinical keratoconus [51]. However, our unpublished data found that the epithelium in patients with subclinical keratoconus had localized thinning of inferior epithelium quantified with minimum thickness. We also found that the epithelium has relative superior thickening by maximum thickness and that standard deviation of epithelial thickness was increased significantly in all regions.

4.3 Keratoconus

Corneas with keratoconus show epithelial remodeling, which minimizes local topographic irregularities and improves corneal curvature [52]. Epithelial thinning precedes other corneal changes in keratoconus [53, 54], and the location of the thinnest zone of the epithelium corresponds with the steepest zone seen on Scheimpflug tomography [10]. Xu et al. reported no significant thinning of the inferior cornea in eyes with keratoconus as compared to normal eyes. However, there was significant thinning of the central epithelium; 53.48 μm in normal eyes and 46.10 μm in eyes with keratoconus [51]. Yadav et al. reported that variation in epithelial thickness across the central 3 mm was significantly larger in eyes with keratoconus. This finding was supported by Pircher et al. who wrote that "epithelial thickness, irregularity, and asymmetry seem to be the most promising diagnostic factors in terms of discriminating between keratoconic eyes and healthy eyes" [55].

4.4 Ocular surface pathology

UHR-OCT can be used for the diagnosis of ocular surface squamous neoplasia (OSSN) and detection of sub-clinical disease [16, 56, 57]. OSSN has several classical features on anterior segment OCT, including thickened, hyper-reflective epithelium with an abrupt transition from normal to abnormal epithelium [16, 57, 58]. The gold standard for diagnosis of OSSN is examination of pathology, but non-invasive methods of diagnosis are helpful as topical chemotherapy becomes increasingly utilized [16]. UHR-OCT provides high-resolution imaging with cross-sectional views; dynamic non-contact scanning modality reduces need for technical expertise compared to UBM and confocal microscopy. However, it has poor penetrance with thicker lesions and cannot reliably detect invasion [16]. UHR-OCT is especially useful as it can non-invasively detect OSSN in the presence of other ocular surface diseases. Co-existing conditions such as mucus membrane pemphigoid or limbal stem cell deficiency make it difficult to diagnosis OSSN based on clinical exam [59].

Corneas with scarring and Salzmann's nodular degeneration have a normal-thickness epithelium overlying a dense, hyper-reflective lesion overlying Bowman's layer on UHR-OCT [16]. Epithelial hypo-reflective cysts without basement membrane thickening are seen in Meesman's dystrophy [60]. Eyes with secondary corneal amyloidosis show deposits of amyloid above Bowman's layer, and destruction of Bowman's layer as the disease progresses [61].

4.5 Physiologic changes after contact lens wear

UHR-OCT can show corneal changes after soft contact lens wear. Epithelial thickness increased by 3.5% and total corneal thickness increased by 10% after 3 hours of patching with soft contact lens wear [62]. Endothelium and Descemet membrane showed no significant change in thickness. Long-term hydrogel lens wearers have been shown to have uniform epithelial thinning [63]. Orthokeratology lenses caused the central epithelium to thin in vertical and horizontal meridians, while the mid-peripheral nasal and temporal epithelium became thicker and the superior mid-peripheral epithelium became thinner. Bowman's layer showed no change from orthokeratology lenses [64].

4.6 Monitoring corneal epithelial defects

UHR-OCT is a useful way to monitor corneal epithelial healing as it provides an objective and three-dimensional evaluation [65]. Corneal wound healing was assessed after epithelial-off corneal collagen cross-linking, and it was noted that epithelium surrounding the fluorescein stained abrasion was not fully settled to the underlying basement membrane [10, 65]. UHR-OCT can also help monitor corneal epithelial healing under a bandage contact lens and can determine the appropriate time for lens removal after pterygium excision [11].

4.7 Post-operative monitoring

UHR-OCT revealed a significant correlation between epithelial thickening and the extent of refractive correction after myopic small incision lenticule extraction. Epithelial thickening of approximately 10% was observed during the first six postoperative months and stabilized after 3 months [66]. Epithelial thickness in eyes treated with photorefractive keratectomy was significantly higher than that of normal eyes at (68.2 vs. 55.8 μm) [24]. This difference was thought to be caused by non-uniformly altered Bowman's layer [24].

Rocha et al. reported a reduction in peripheral epithelial thickness and decreased regional variation in epithelial thickness consistent with increased corneal curvature after corneal collagen crosslinking [52]. UHR-OCT of corneal wound healing after epithelial-off cross-linking correlated well with fluorescein photographs and visualized the stromal demarcation line [65]. Most of the data about the demarcation line seen in cross-linking comes from use of the SD-OCT and further research is needed [67].

Zarei-Ghanavati et al. showed that epithelium covers the Boston type I keratoprosthesis edge and seals the potential space in the interface. They proposed that failure to epithelialize this interface and lack of epithelial sealing around the keratoprosthesis edge might be associated with endophthalmitis [68].

5. Bowman's membrane pathology

5.1 Subclinical keratoconus

Vertical thickness of Bowman's layer in subclinical keratoconus was decreased inferiorly compared with normal control eyes [51]. Our group demonstrated that Bowman's layer in patients with subclinical keratoconus was significantly thinner centrally and inferiorly, and could be quantified with mean thickness, minimum thickness, Bowman's ectasia index and Bowman's ectasia index-max [69].

5.2 Keratoconus

Bowman's layer shows thinning, disintegration and breakage on pathological specimens of eyes with keratoconus (**Figure 2**). Histopathological light and electron microscopy studies of these eyes can be helpful for the diagnosis of keratoconus [70]. Interestingly, these changes happen before stromal changes [71]. Abou Shousha et al. demonstrated that vertical topographic thickness maps of keratoconus patients had characteristic localized relative inferior thinning of Bowman's layer. Inferior average thickness, inferior minimum thickness, Bowman's ectasia index and Bowman's ectasia index-max were all correlated with the severity of keratoconus. The inferior average thickness of Bowman's layer in eyes with keratoconus was 12 μm compared with 15 μm in normal eyes [72]. Light scatter from Bowman's layer in eyes with keratoconus was significantly higher but did not correlate with disease severity [13].

5.3 Corneal and ocular surface pathology

UHR-OCT can detect early secondary corneal amyloidosis as a dense spot in Bowman's layer [61]. Corneas with Thiel-Behnke Dystrophy have extensive deposits of hyper-reflective material in a saw-tooth pattern on the surface of Bowman's layer [60]. UHR-OCT images may become adjunct to clinical evaluation and provide an optical biopsy image in other conditions. Eyes with spheroidal degeneration show cystic structures in Bowman's layer and superficial stroma, and Salzmann's nodular degeneration has hyper-reflective material which replaces anterior stroma and Bowman's layer with thin epithelium [60] (**Figure 2**). Limbal stem cell deficiency exhibits a hyper-reflective material which replaces Bowman's layer as well as the anterior stroma, with irregular overlying epithelium (**Figure 3**).

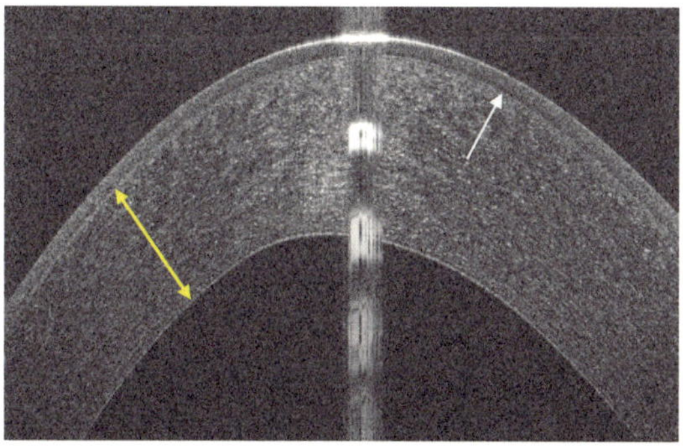

Figure 2.
A prototypical cross-sectional UHR-OCT image of a human cornea with keratoconus; focal disintegration of Bowman's layer (white arrow), focal stromal thinning (yellow arrow).

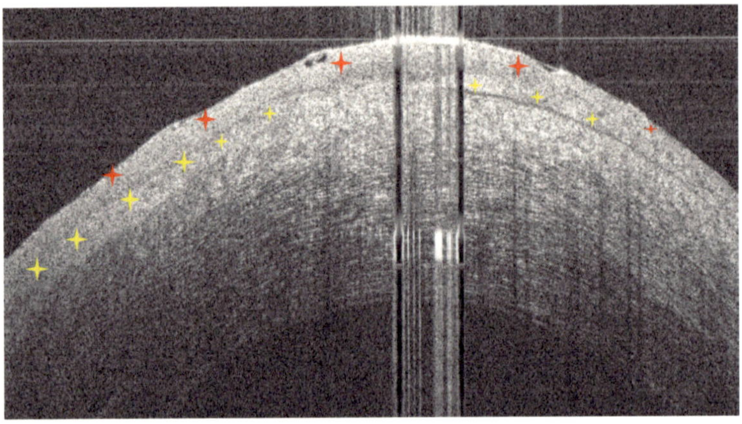

Figure 3.
A prototypical cross-sectional UHR-OCT image of a human cornea with Limbal stem cell deficiency; a hyper-reflective material (yellow stars) which replaces anterior stroma and Bowman's layer with irregular overlying epithelium (red stars).

5.4 Eyes after refractive surgery

Bowman's layer significantly decreases in eyes after photorefractive keratectomy, and was on average 14.0 μm compared with normal eyes at 18.7 μm. There is significant variability after photorefractive keratectomy with some regions thicker than in normal eyes but most much thinner. The procedure also causes uneven epithelial thickness [24].

6. Corneal pathology within stroma

6.1 Corneal inflammatory and infectious diseases

UHR-OCT can help with the diagnosis of Acanthamoeba and herpetic keratitis. Acanthamoeba cysts show up are seen as highly reflective dots in the stroma and radial keratoneuritis presents as thickening of the corneal nerves with ragged borders [10]. In post-herpetic keratitis corneas, UHR-OCT shows corneal thinning with areas of calcification and lipid deposition as single highly reflective scattering zones. Corneal neovascularization also appears as a hypo-reflective zone [10].

UHR-OCT is especially useful for assessment of corneal thinning in cases of impending perforation. Rodriguez et al. evaluated the use of UHR-OCT in the differentiation of inflammatory versus non-inflammatory, such as Terrien Marginal Degeneration, causes of peripheral corneal thinning. In the inflammatory group, UHR-OCT revealed a hyper-reflective subepithelial band in the area of thinning, which was not seen in Terrien marginal degeneration [73].

6.2 Stromal corneal dystrophies

UHR-OCT can evaluate the depth of deposits in stromal corneal dystrophies, which can be used to guide surgical therapy. Eyes with granular dystrophy show hyper-reflective material in the anterior stroma and clear intervening spaces. Macular dystrophy corneas show hyper-reflective stroma with areas of discrete, small hyper-reflective deposits in the subepithelial space, stroma, and Descemet's membrane [60].

6.3 Refractive surgery

UHR-OCT can be used to analyze the integrity of the corneal flap. High resolution structural characteristics of the opaque bubble layer can predict incomplete lamellar flap dissections. The opaque bubble layer can also be seen to extend anterior to the flap dissection plane up to Bowman's membrane [74]. UHR-OCT can also image progression of flap melt and epithelial ingrowth [2].

6.4 Subclinical keratoconus

Xu et al. reported that stromal vertical thickness profiles in eyes with subclinical keratoconus were thinner inferiorly compared with normal eyes [51]. Another group showed focal inferotemporal thinning, slightly more inferior than temporal. However, the degree of relative thinning was not as significant as on the epithelial pattern deviation map [75].

6.5 Keratoconus

Eyes with keratoconus had a thinner stromal thickness than normal eyes for the entire vertical meridian profile. In the keratoconus group, the thinnest central stromal thickness was 383.8 μm [51]. Sandali et al. used Fourier-domain OCT to create a reproducible classification scheme for patient with keratoconus [76]. Fuentes et al. used Fourier-domain OCT (5 mm of axial resolution) to look for risk factors for hydrops in advanced keratoconus. They revealed that features such as increased epithelial thickness, Bowman's layer hyper-reflection, and stromal thinning at the cone may be associated with increased risk [77]. UHR-OCT is also useful to identify depth of crosslinking (**Figure 4**). However, Rocha et al. demonstrated that there were no significant differences in regional stromal thickness profiles at any corneal location after corneal collagen crosslinking for eyes with either keratoconus or postoperative corneal ectasia [52].

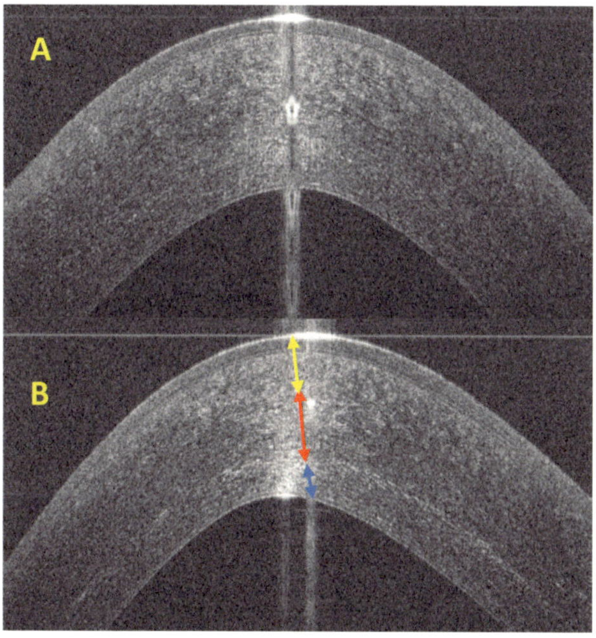

Figure 4.
Prototypical cross-sectional UHR-OCT images of keratoconus before (a) and 1 month after collagen cross-linking (B); cross-linking demarcation band thickness (red arrow), depth (yellow arrow), and base (blue arrow).

7. Corneal pathology within endothelium/Descemet membrane complex (En/DM)

7.1 Fuchs' endothelial corneal dystrophy

Abou Shousha et al. published UHR-OCT characteristics of Fuchs' dystrophy patients. Descemet membrane appeared as a thickened band with two opaque lines; the anterior line was smooth while the posterior line was wavy and irregular with areas of focal thickening (**Figure 5**) [9]. Descemet membrane thickness was increased in Fuchs' dystrophy patients compared with normal subjects [9].

7.2 Detection of corneal graft rejection

Basement membrane thickening has previously been established as evidence of graft rejection in solid organs transplantation [78, 79]. Abou Shousha et al. demonstrated that thickening of the En/DM also occurs in corneal graft rejection (**Figure 6**) [80]. This study was limited by the resolution of HD-OCT as it was not possible to differentiate

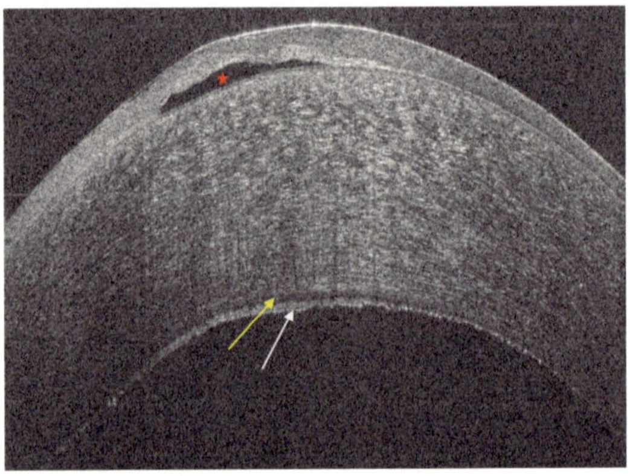

Figure 5.
A prototypical cross-sectional UHR-OCT image of a human cornea with Fuchs' endothelial dystrophy; sub-epithelial vesicle (red star), Descemet membrane appeared as a thickened band with two opaque lines; the anterior line (yellow arrow) was smooth while the posterior line (white arrow) was wavy and irregular with areas of focal thickening.

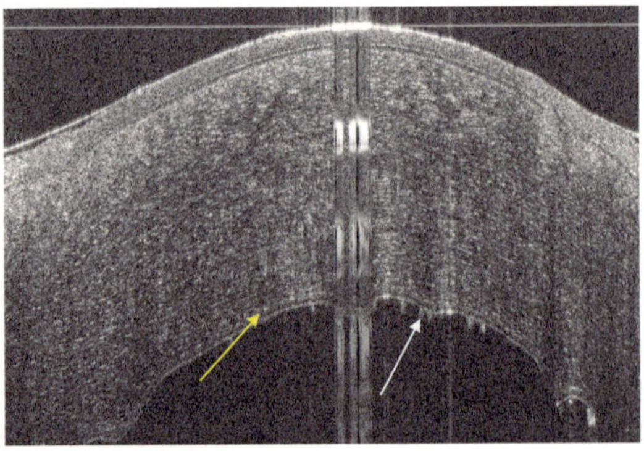

Figure 6.
A prototypical cross-sectional UHR-OCT image of a full thickness corneal transplant with active rejection: Descemet membrane appeared as a thickened band with two hyper-reflective lines; the anterior line (yellow arrow) was smooth while the posterior line (white arrow) was wavy, broader with occasional nodular excrescences.

between Descemet membrane, endothelium, and a potential retro-corneal membrane. Subsequent *ex vivo* data revealed that Descemet membrane is responsible for thickening of the En/DM complex in rejected corneal grafts [30].

7.3. Monitoring surgical patients

Transient corneal edema seen after phacoemulsification was caused by changes in the central corneal thickness, stroma and En/DM complex. There were no significant post-operative changes in Bowman's layer or epithelium. Pre-operative En/DM thickness may indicate the integrity of the endothelium and could be used to predict endothelial cell loss after phacoemulsification [81].

8. Corneal graft screening

Donor tissue quality is critical in the outcome of corneal transplantation [82]. Specular microscopy is the current gold standard for corneal graft screening, but only evaluates the health of the endothelium. We do not currently have an efficient method to screen for epithelial and stromal pathology such as prior refractive surgery, keratoconus or stromal opacities [82]. UHR-OCT can evaluate response to tissue processing in lamellar keratoplasty by revealing interface debris and cavitation bubbles after treatment with femtosecond laser, which may be used to correlate with post-operative outcomes [83]. Our unpublished data demonstrated the use of UHR-OCT to measure the En/DM complex thickness in donor corneas in a sterile container, and has promising results to screen grafts for early endothelial changes [84].

9. Future directions

Future developments include clinical application of the technique to screen donor corneas before transplantation. The newest generation of imaging, micro-OCT (μOCT), uses an isotropic spatial resolution of 1–2 μm. It can detect key cellular and subcellular components such as keratocytes, collagen fibers and corneal nerves. This new technology has the potential to improve our understanding of corneal anatomy and disease.

10. Conclusions

UHR-OCT of the anterior segment enables us to perform an optical biopsy of the tear film and all layers in the cornea in normal subjects and those with pathology. These advancements provide understanding about pathological changes in microlayers of the cornea. The main advantages of the OCT include the rapid, non-invasive, in vivo imaging of structures with quantitative measurements. Recent improvements in OCT technology have led to an increase in clinical and research applications. Novel developments, such as the new-generation micro-OCT and artificial intelligence, have the potential to revolutionize corneal disease diagnosis and classifications.

Conflict of interest

Vatookarn Roongpoovapatr, Jane Cook and Taher K. Eleiwa—None to declare.

Sonia H. Yoo and Mohamed Abou Shousha—.

Financial Support: This study was supported by a NEI K23 award (K23EY026118), NEI core center grant to the University of Miami (P30 EY014801), and Research to Prevent Blindness (RPB).

The funding organization had no role in the design or conduct of this research.

Conflict of Interest: United States Non-Provisional Patents (Application No. 8992023 and 61809518), and PCT/US2018/013409. Patents and PCT are owned by University of Miami and licensed to Resolve Ophthalmics, LLC. Mohamed Abou Shousha is an equity holder and sits on the Board of Directors for Resolve Ophthalmics, LLC.

Sonia Yoo is a co-inventor of intellectual property used in the study.

Author details

Vatookarn Roongpoovapatr[1,2], Jane C. Cook[1*], Taher K. Eleiwa[1,3], Sonia H. Yoo[1] and Mohamed Abou Shousha[1]

1 Miller School of Medicine, Bascom Palmer Eye Institute, University of Miami, Miami, FL, United States

2 Department of Ophthalmology, Mettapracharak (Wat Raikhing) Hospital, Nakorn-Pathom, Thailand

3 Department of Ophthalmology, Faculty of Medicine, Benha University, Egypt

*Address all correspondence to: janecatycook@gmail.com

References

[1] Ang M, Baskaran M, Werkmeister RM, et al. Anterior segment optical coherence tomography. Progress in Retinal and Eye Research. 2018;**66**:132-156

[2] Wang J, Abou Shousha M, Perez VL, et al. Ultra-high resolution optical coherence tomography for imaging the anterior segment of the eye. Ophthalmic Surgery, Lasers & Imaging. 2011;**42** (Suppl):S15-S27

[3] Bajwa A, Aman R, Reddy AK. A comprehensive review of diagnostic imaging technologies to evaluate the retina and the optic disk. International Ophthalmology. 2015;**35**:733-755

[4] Han SB, Liu Y-C, Noriega KM, Mehta JS. Applications of anterior segment optical coherence tomography in cornea and ocular surface diseases. Journal of Ophthalmology. 2016:4971572

[5] Maeda N. Optical coherence tomography for corneal diseases. Eye & Contact Lens. 2010;**36**:254-259

[6] Huo T, Wang C, Zhang X, et al. Ultrahigh-speed optical coherence tomography utilizing all-optical 40 MHz swept-source. Journal of Biomedical Optics. 2015;**20**:030503

[7] Kolb JP, Klein T, Kufner CL, et al. Ultra-widefield retinal MHz-OCT imaging with up to 100 degrees viewing angle. Biomedical Optics Express. 2015;**6**:1534-1552

[8] Zhi Z, Qin W, Wang J, et al. 4D optical coherence tomography-based micro-angiography achieved by 1.6-MHz FDML swept source. Optics Letters. 2015;**40**:1779-1782

[9] Shousha MA, Perez VL, Wang J, et al. Use of ultra-high-resolution optical coherence tomography to detect in vivo characteristics of Descemet's membrane in Fuchs' dystrophy. Ophthalmology. 2010;**117**:1220-1227

[10] Werkmeister RM, Sapeta S, Schmidl D, et al. Ultrahigh-resolution OCT imaging of the human cornea. Biomedical Optics Express. 2017;**8**:1221-1239

[11] Chen D, Lian Y, Li J, et al. Monitor corneal epithelial healing under bandage contact lens using ultrahigh-resolution optical coherence tomography after pterygium surgery. Eye & Contact Lens. 2014;**40**:175-180

[12] Cui L, Wang J, Perez VL, et al. Visualization of the precorneal tear film using ultrahigh resolution optical coherence tomography in dry eye. Eye & Contact Lens. 2012;**38**:240-244

[13] Yadav R, Kottaiyan R, Ahmad K, Yoon G. Epithelium and Bowman's layer thickness and light scatter in keratoconic cornea evaluated using ultrahigh resolution optical coherence tomography. Journal of Biomedical Optics. 2012;**17**(11):116010

[14] Huang D, Swanson EA, Lin CP, et al. Optical coherence tomography. Science. 1991;**254**:1178-1181

[15] Qazi Y, Aggarwal S, Hamrah P. Image-guided evaluation and monitoring of treatment response in patients with dry eye disease. Graefe's Archive for Clinical and Experimental Ophthalmology. 2014;**252**:857-872

[16] Thomas BJ, Galor A, Nanji AA, et al. Ultra high-resolution anterior segment optical coherence tomography in the diagnosis and management of ocular surface squamous neoplasia. The Ocular Surface. 2014;**12**:46-58

[17] Drexler W. Ultrahigh-resolution optical coherence tomography. Journal of Biomedical Optics. 2004;**9**:47-74

[18] Chen Q, Wang J, Tao A, et al. Ultrahigh-resolution measurement by optical coherence tomography of dynamic tear film changes on contact lenses. Investigative Ophthalmology & Visual Science. 2010;**51**:1988-1993

[19] Chen J, Lee L. Clinical applications and new developments of optical coherence tomography: An evidence-based review. Clinical & Experimental Optometry. 2007;**90**:317-335

[20] Sridhar MS. Anatomy of cornea and ocular surface. Indian Journal of Ophthalmology. 2018;**66**:190-194

[21] Feizi S, Jafarinasab MR, Karimian F, et al. Central and peripheral corneal thickness measurement in normal and keratoconic eyes using three corneal pachymeters. J. Ophthalmic Vis. Res. 2014;**9**:296-304

[22] Meek KM, Fullwood NJ. Corneal and scleral collagens- a microscopist's perspective. Micron. 2001;**32**:261-272

[23] Dua HS, Faraj LA, Said DG, et al. Human corneal anatomy redefined: A novel pre-Descemet's layer (Dua's layer). Ophthalmology. 2013;**120**:1778-1785

[24] Werkmeister RM, Alex A, Kaya S, et al. Measurement of tear film thickness using ultrahigh-resolution optical coherence tomography. Investigative Ophthalmology & Visual Science. 2013;**54**:5578-5583

[25] Wang J, Aquavella J, Palakuru J, et al. Relationships between central tear film thickness and tear menisci of the upper and lower eyelids. Investigative Ophthalmology & Visual Science. 2006;**47**:4349-4355

[26] Schmoll T, Unterhuber A, Kolbitsch C, et al. Precise thickness measurements of Bowman's layer, epithelium, and tear film. Optometry and Vision Science. 2012;**89**:E795-E802

[27] Dos Santos VA, Schmetterer L, Triggs GJ, et al. Super-resolved thickness maps of thin film phantoms and in vivo visualization of tear film lipid layer using OCT. Biomedical Optics Express. 2016;**7**:2650-2670

[28] Francoz M, Karamoko I, Baudouin C, Labbé A. Ocular surface epithelial thickness evaluation with spectral-domain optical coherence tomography. Investigative Ophthalmology & Visual Science. 2011;**52**:9116-9123

[29] Niederer RL, Perumal D, Sherwin T, McGhee CNJ. Age-related differences in the normal human cornea: A laser scanning in vivo confocal microscopy study. The British Journal of Ophthalmology. 2007;**91**:1165-1169

[30] Du C, Wang J, Cui L, et al. Vertical and horizontal corneal epithelial thickness profiles determined by ultrahigh resolution optical coherence tomography. Cornea. 2012;**31**:1036-1043

[31] Tao A, Wang J, Chen Q, et al. Topographic thickness of Bowman's layer determined by ultra-high resolution spectral domain-optical coherence tomography. Investigative Ophthalmology & Visual Science. 2011;**52**:3901-3907

[32] VanDenBerg R, Diakonis VF, Bozung A, et al. Descemet membrane thickening as a sign for the diagnosis of corneal graft rejection: An ex vivo study. Cornea. 2017;**36**:1535-1537

[33] Bizheva K, Haines L, Mason E, et al. In vivo imaging and morphometry of the human pre-Descemet's layer and endothelium with ultrahigh-resolution optical coherence tomography. Investigative Ophthalmology & Visual Science. 2016;**57**:2782-2787

[34] Wolffsohn JS, Arita R, Chalmers R, et al. TFOS DEWS II diagnostic methodology report. The Ocular Surface. 2017;**15**:539-574

[35] Craig JP, Nelson JD, Azar DT, et al. TFOS DEWS II report executive summary. The Ocular Surface. 2017;**15**:802-812

[36] Wang J, Palakuru JR, Aquavella JV. Correlations among upper and lower tear menisci, noninvasive tear break-up time, and the Schirmer test. American Journal of Ophthalmology. 2008;**145**:795-800

[37] Li J, Shen M, Wang J, et al. Clinical significance of tear menisci in dry eye. Eye & Contact Lens. 2012;**38**:183-187

[38] Tittler EH, Bujak MC, Nguyen P, et al. Between-grader repeatability of tear meniscus measurements using Fourier-domain OCT in patients with dry eye. Ophthalmic Surgery, Lasers & Imaging. 2011;**42**:423-427

[39] Schmidl D, Schmetterer L, Witkowska KJ, et al. Tear film thickness after treatment with artificial tears in patients with moderate dry eye disease. Cornea. 2015;**34**:421-426

[40] Wozniak PA, Schmidl D, Bata AM, et al. Effect of different lubricant eye gels on tear film thickness as measured with ultrahigh-resolution optical coherence tomography. Acta Ophthalmologica. 2017;**95**:e307-e313

[41] Kaya S, Schmidl D, Schmetterer L, et al. Effect of hyaluronic acid on tear film thickness as assessed with ultra-high resolution optical coherence tomography. Acta Ophthalmologica. 2015;**93**:439-443

[42] Li M, Wang J, Shen M, et al. Effect of punctal occlusion on tear menisci in symptomatic contact lens wearers. Cornea. 2012;**31**:1014-1022

[43] Cui L, Shen M, Wang MR, Wang J. Micrometer-scale contact lens movements imaged by ultrahigh-resolution optical coherence tomography. American Journal of Ophthalmology. 2012;**153**:275-283.e1

[44] Cui L, Chen S, Zhou W, et al. Characterization of soft contact Lens edge fitting during daily Wear using ultrahigh-resolution optical coherence tomography. Journal of Ophthalmology. 2018;**3463595**:1-7

[45] Wang J, Jiao S, Ruggeri M, et al. In situ visualization of tears on contact lens using ultra high resolution optical coherence tomography. Eye & Contact Lens. 2009;**35**:44-49

[46] Çakır B, Doğan E, Çelik E, et al. Effects of artificial tear treatment on corneal epithelial thickness and corneal topography findings in dry eye patients. Journal Français d'Ophtalmologie. 2018;**41**:407-411

[47] Erdélyi B, Kraak R, Zhivov A, et al. In vivo confocal laser scanning microscopy of the cornea in dry eye. Graefe's Archive for Clinical and Experimental Ophthalmology. 2007;**245**:39-44

[48] Villani E, Galimberti D, Viola F, et al. The cornea in Sjogren's syndrome: An in vivo confocal study. Investigative Ophthalmology & Visual Science. 2007;**48**:2017-2022

[49] El-Fayoumi D, Youssef MM, Khafagy MM, et al. Assessment of corneal and tear film parameters in rheumatoid arthritis patients using anterior segment spectral domain optical coherence tomography. Ocular Immunology and Inflammation. 2018;**26**:632-638

[50] Tuominen ISJ, Konttinen YT, Vesaluoma MH, et al. Corneal innervation and morphology in primary Sjögren's syndrome. Investigative Ophthalmology & Visual Science. 2003;**44**:2545-2549

[51] Kanellopoulos AJ, Asimellis G. In vivo 3-dimensional corneal epithelial thickness mapping as an indicator of dry eye: Preliminary clinical assessment.

American Journal of Ophthalmology. 2014;**57**:63-68.e2

[52] Xu Z, Jiang J, Yang C, et al. Value of corneal epithelial and Bowman's layer vertical thickness profiles generated by UHR-OCT for sub-clinical keratoconus diagnosis. Scientific Reports. 2016;**6**:31550

[53] Rocha KM, Rocha KM, Perez-Straziota CE, et al. Epithelial and stromal remodeling after corneal collagen cross-linking evaluated by spectral-domain OCT. Journal of Refractive Surgery. 2014;**30**:122-127

[54] Catalan S, Cadarso L, Esteves F, et al. Assessment of corneal epithelial thickness in asymmetric keratoconic eyes and normal eyes using Fourier domain optical coherence tomography. Journal of Ophthalmology. 2016;**5697343**:1-7

[55] Temstet C, Sandali O, Bouheraoua N, et al. Corneal epithelial thickness mapping using Fourier-domain optical coherence tomography for detection of form fruste keratoconus. Journal of Cataract and Refractive Surgery. 2015;**41**:812-820

[56] Pircher N, Schwarzhans F, Holzer S, et al. Distinguishing keratoconic eyes and healthy eyes using ultrahigh-resolution optical coherence tomography-based corneal epithelium thickness mapping. American Journal of Ophthalmology. 2018;**189**:47-54

[57] Medina CA, Plesec T, Singh AD. Optical coherence tomography imaging of ocular and periocular tumours. The British Journal of Ophthalmology. 2014;**98**(Suppl 2):ii40-ii46

[58] Shousha MA, Karp CL, Perez VL, et al. Diagnosis and management of conjunctival and corneal intraepithelial neoplasia using ultra high-resolution optical coherence tomography. Ophthalmology. 2011;**118**:1531-1537

[59] Shousha MA, Karp CL, Canto AP, et al. Diagnosis of ocular surface lesions using ultra-high-resolution optical coherence tomography. Ophthalmology. 2013;**120**:883-891

[60] Ong SS, Vora GK, Gupta PK. Anterior segment imaging in ocular surface squamous neoplasia. Journal of Ophthalmology. 2016;**5435092**:1-12

[61] Atallah M, Joag M, Galor A, et al. Role of high resolution optical coherence tomography in diagnosing ocular surface squamous neoplasia with coexisting ocular surface diseases. The Ocular Surface. 2017;**15**:688-695

[62] Vajzovic LM, Karp CL, Haft P, et al. Ultra high-resolution anterior segment optical coherence tomography in the evaluation of anterior corneal dystrophies and degenerations. Ophthalmology. 2011;**118**:1291-1296

[63] Araki-Sasaki K, Osakabe Y, Fukuoka H, et al. Findings of secondary corneal amyloidosis with ultrahigh-resolution optical coherence tomography. Clinical Ophthalmology. 2014;**8**:2115-2119

[64] Hutchings N, Simpson TL, Hyun C, et al. Swelling of the human cornea revealed by high-speed, ultrahigh-resolution optical coherence tomography. Investigative Ophthalmology & Visual Science. 2010;**51**:4579-4584

[65] Pérez JG, Méijome JMG, Jalbert I, et al. Corneal epithelial thinning profile induced by long-term wear of hydrogel lenses. Cornea. 2003;**22**:304-307

[66] Lian Y, Shen M, Jiang J, et al. Vertical and horizontal thickness profiles of the corneal epithelium and Bowman's layer after orthokeratology. Investigative Ophthalmology & Visual Science. 2013;**54**:691-696

[67] Bata AM, Witkowska KJ, Wozniak PA, et al. Effect of a matrix therapy

agent on corneal epithelial healing after standard collagen cross-linking in patients with keratoconus: A randomized clinical trial. JAMA Ophthalmology. 2016;**134**:1169-1176

[68] Luft N, Ring MH, Dirisamer M, et al. Corneal epithelial remodeling induced by small incision lenticule extraction (SMILE). Investigative Ophthalmology & Visual Science. 2016;**57**:OCT176-OCT183

[69] Kanellopoulos AJ, Asimellis G. Epithelial remodeling after partial topography-guided normalization and high-fluence short-duration crosslinking (Athens protocol): Results up to 1 year. Journal of Cataract and Refractive Surgery. 2014;**40**:1597-1602

[70] Zarei-Ghanavati S, Betancurt C, Mas AM, et al. Ultra high resolution optical coherence tomography in Boston type I keratoprosthesis. J. Ophthalmic Vis. Res. 2015;**10**:26-32

[71] Sykakis E, Carley F, Irion L, et al. An in depth analysis of histopathological characteristics found in keratoconus. Pathology. 2012;**44**:234-239

[72] Tuori AJ, Virtanen I, Aine E, et al. The immunohistochemical composition of corneal basement membrane in keratoconus. Current Eye Research. 1997;**16**:792-801

[73] Abou Shousha M, Perez VL, Fraga Santini Canto AP, et al. The use of Bowman's layer vertical topographic thickness map in the diagnosis of keratoconus. Ophthalmology. 2014;**121**:988-993

[74] Rodriguez M, Yesilirmak N, Chhadva P, et al. High-resolution optical coherence tomography in the differentiation of inflammatory versus noninflammatory peripheral corneal thinning. Cornea. 2017;**36**:48-52

[75] Hurmeric V, Yoo SH, Fishler J, et al. In vivo structural characteristics of the femtosecond LASIK-induced opaque bubble layers with ultrahigh-resolution SD-OCT. Ophthalmic Surgery, Lasers & Imaging. 2010;**41**(Suppl):S109-S113

[76] Sandali O, El Sanharawi M, Temstet C, et al. Fourier-domain optical coherence tomography imaging in keratoconus: A corneal structural classification. Ophthalmology. 2013;**120**:2403-2412

[77] Fuentes E, Sandali O, El Sanharawi M, et al. Anatomic predictive factors of acute corneal hydrops in keratoconus. Ophthalmology. 2015;**122**:1653-1659

[78] Liapis G, Singh HK, Derebail VK, et al. Diagnostic significance of peritubular capillary basement membrane multilaminations in kidney allografts: Old concepts revisited. Transplantation. 2012;**94**:620-629

[79] Demetris AJ, Murase N, Lee RG, et al. Chronic rejection. A general overview of histopathology and pathophysiology with emphasis on liver, heart and intestinal allografts. Annals of Transplantation. 1997;**2**:27-44

[80] Abou Shousha M, Yoo SH, Sayed MS, et al. In vivo characteristics of corneal endothelium/Descemet membrane complex for the diagnosis of corneal graft rejection. American Journal of Ophthalmology. 2017;**178**:27-37

[81] Tao A, Chen Z, Shao Y, et al. Phacoemulsification induced transient swelling of corneal Descemet's endothelium complex imaged with ultra-high resolution optical coherence tomography. PLoS One. 2013;**8**:e80986

[82] Ghouali W, Grieve K, Bellefqih S, et al. Full-field optical coherence tomography of human donor and pathological corneas. Current Eye Research. 2015;**40**:526-534

[83] Brown JS, Wang D, Li X, et al. In situ ultrahigh-resolution optical coherence tomography characterization of eye bank corneal tissue processed for lamellar keratoplasty. Cornea. 2008;**27**:802-810

[84] Chen S, Liu X, Wang N, et al. Visualizing micro-anatomical structures of the posterior cornea with micro-optical coherence tomography. Scientific Reports. 2017;**7**:10752

Chapter 2

Clinical Application of Optical Coherence Tomography in the Corneal Degenerations

Constanza Caramello Álvarez, María A. del Buey, Paula Casas, Sara Marco, Enrique Mínguez and Francisco J. Ascaso

Abstract

Anterior segment optical coherence tomography (**AS-OCT**) has become an essential tool in the diagnosis and management of corneal degenerations. AS-OCT optical findings and thickness measurements are useful for the proper evaluation of the ocular surface diseases. AS-OCT imaging provides noninvasive information necessary to decide clinical and surgical management. This device helps to achieve a correct pre-intervention investigation and will allow physicians to compare the corneal status after the surgical process. Thus, it is useful to evaluate the corneal thickness, areas of hyper-reflective material, and corneal fibrosis in certain disorders such as **Salzmann's nodular degeneration** (**SND**) and **Terrien's marginal degeneration** (**TMD**), before and following the surgical process.

Keywords: anterior segment optical coherence tomography, corneal degenerations, Salzmann's nodular degeneration, Terrien's marginal degeneration, Dellen, band keratopathy, ocular surface disease, keratoplasty, lamellar keratoplasty

1. Introduction

Optical coherence tomography (**OCT**) was developed to assess the ocular posterior segment. **Anterior segment OCT** (**AS-OCT**) was not described until 1994, and the first AS-OCT device was commercialized in 2005 [1–3].

The improvement from time domain to spectral domain OCT allowed higher axial resolution images. AS-OCT devices can achieve high-resolution imaging, ranging from less than 5 μm (ultra-high-resolution) to greater than 5 μm (high-resolution), providing a noninvasive, in vivo, cross-sectional image of the ocular surface and corneal structure [4, 5].

Spectral domain OCT (SD-OCT) devices include the **Spectralis® HRA + OCT system (Heidelberg Engineering GmbH, Germany).** It can achieve 40,000 A-scans/second and has a 3.9–7 μm axial resolution, a 14 μm transverse resolution, a 1.9 mm scan depth, and an 870 nm average wavelength [4–6]. This AS-OCT device has been used to capture the corneal OCT images showed along this chapter (**Figure 1**).

AS-OCT is clinically useful for the examination, diagnosis, and management of most of the anterior segment pathologies [4, 7–9] (**Figure 2**). Additionally, it is

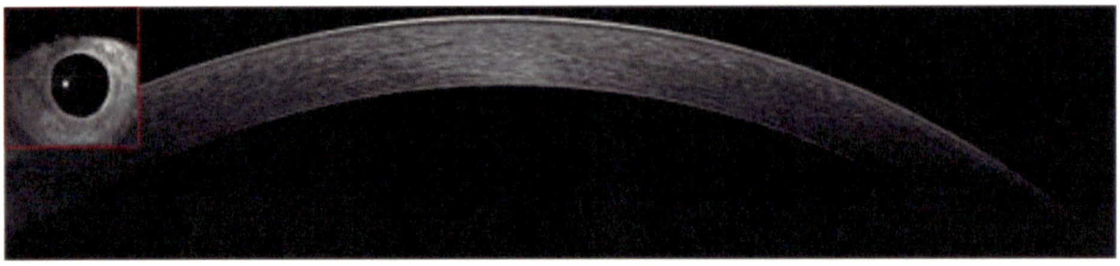

Figure 1.
Corneal AS-OCT imaging from Heidelberg Spectralis OCT system. The corneal AS-OCT image displays a normal corneal tissue. The layers with the highest hyper-reflectivity are the anterior surface of the cornea and the posterior limit of the cornea with the anterior chamber. The stroma appears as a large band of variable intensity, increasing the signal in the apical zone, due to the perpendicular impact of light reflection on the disposition of collagen fibers.

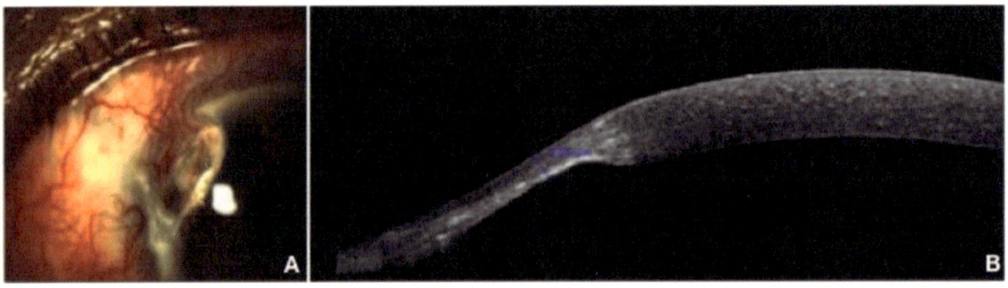

Figure 2.
(A) Anterior segment (AS) slit-lamp biomicroscopy shows a corneal Dellen due to a previous pterygium surgery: the perilimbar elevation produces an inadequate hydration of the adjacent cornea. (B) Corneal AS-OCT imaging demonstrates a thinning peripheral zone. This thinning area can be measured, and periodic controls can be made by AS-OCT.

helpful for planning and performing surgery as well as monitoring postoperative cares [1]. AS-OCT imaging requires no contact, which prevents patient discomfort and image distortion. The development of axial resolution, the improvement in scans speeds, and the deeper tissue penetrance allow corneal AS-OCT to recognize structural details in the corneal epithelium, stroma, and conjunctiva, allowing a characterization of corneal disorders [9].

Clinical evaluation and anterior segment (AS) slit-lamp biomicroscopy exam are still the first step in the diagnosis of corneal pathologies and cannot be replaced by corneal AS-OCT images. This technique has to be used as an adjunctive tool, especially in cases in which the diagnosis is clinically equivocal [4, 10]. Corneal AS-OCT imaging has shown to be useful helping to decide the pathology management and to assess the disease resolution. Unfortunately, in some corneal diseases, a histopathologic corneal exam will be necessary to confirm the diagnosis [10].

Corneal AS-OCT imaging can provide optical diagnostic signs for some specific corneal disorders [11]. Thus, corneal hyper-reflectivity can be defined as an increased whiteness compared to corneal tissue of the same location seen in normal subjects, whereas corneal hypo-reflectivity can be defined as an increased darkness compared to corneal tissue of the same location seen in normal individuals [10] (**Figures 2** and **3**). In cases of pathological cornea, a variable increase in reflectivity can be found in case of scars, edema, fibrosis, or material deposits. An attenuated signal is shown in case of fluid accumulation and cystic lesions [10]. In certain cases, AS slit-lamp biomicroscopy evaluation is not able to differentiate an inflammatory disorder from a degenerative disease. In patients with clinical history of inflammation and corneal thinning, corneal AS-OCT imaging shows a hyper-reflective band under the corneal epithelium in the area of thinning, which is not

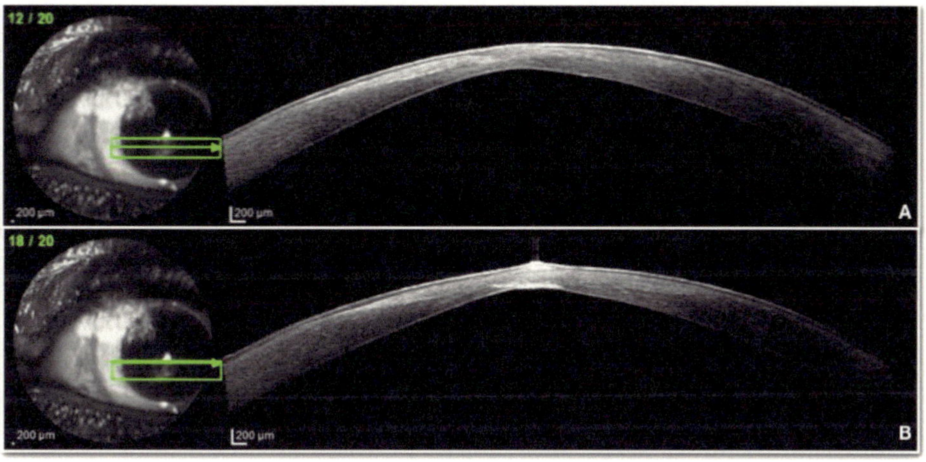

Figure 3.
(A and B) Corneal AS-OCT imaging from the Heidelberg Spectralis OCT device. The image demonstrated a thinning central corneal area with a hyper-reflective signal. The hyper-reflective zone is due to a subepithelial, anterior stroma and endothelial fibrosis.

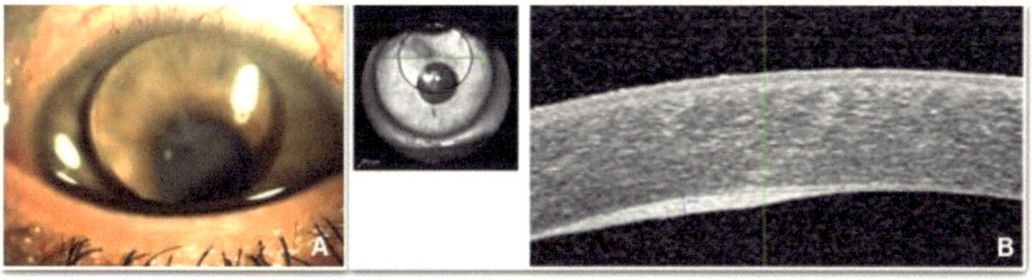

Figure 4.
(A) AS slit-lamp evaluation showing a silicone bubble in the anterior chamber following a retinal detachment surgery. (B) Corneal AS-OCT analysis demonstrated a corneal posterior hyper-reflective zone and fibrosis. The corneal fibrosis area is caused by the silicone direct damage in the endothelial cells.

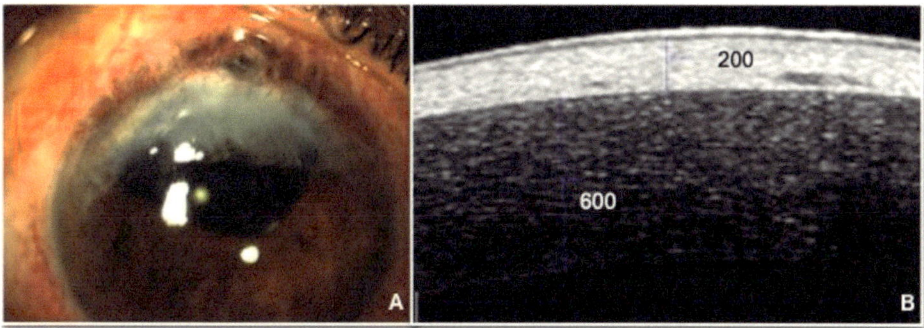

Figure 5.
(A) AS slit-lamp examination showing a corneal superior opacity with iris incarceration due to a previous retinal detachment and a complicated cataract surgery. (B) AS-OCT imaging demonstrated a hyper-reflective and fibrotic area. The opacified zone can be measured by the Heidelberg Spectralis OCT caliper tool.

seen in patients with noninflammatory melts and thinning [4]. This phenomenon can be helpful to achieve a correct management of corneal pathologies (**Figure 4**).

Corneal AS-OCT imaging is also useful for the measurements of corneal scar depth [1] (**Figure 5**). It has demonstrated to be able to define the rim of a corneal opacity

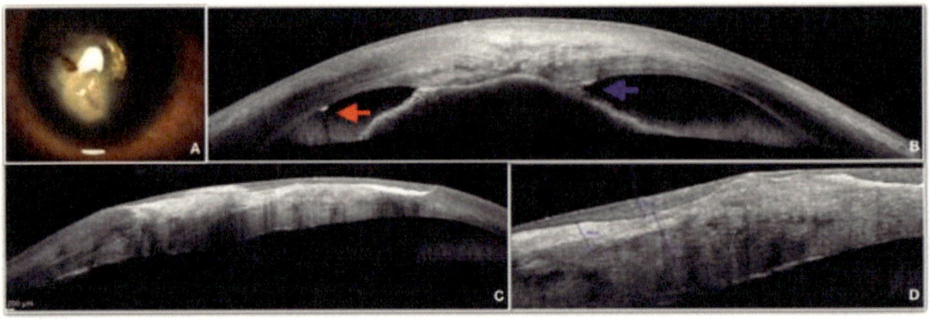

Figure 6.
(A) AS slit-lamp biomicroscopy demonstrates a central and deep corneal opacification due to a traumatic perforation in a child. (B) AS-OCT evaluation shows a strange foreign body in the corneal endothelium (red arrow). The iris is incarcerated in the posterior corneal layers because of the perforating traumatism (blue arrow). (C) AS-OCT imaging displays an irregular stroma with hyper-reflective zones in the fibrosis areas. (D) The caliper tool can measure the respective corneal areas helping the physician to achieve a correct surgical management.

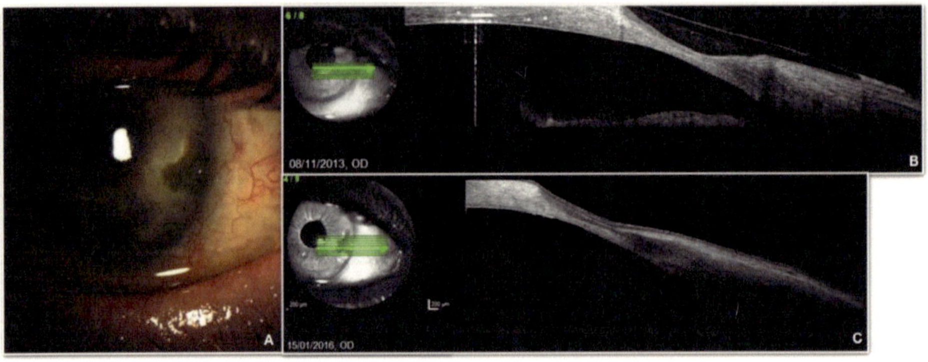

Figure 7.
(A) AS slit-lamp evaluation shows a corneal Dellen due to a previous pterygium surgery in the peripheral nasal area. (A, B) AS-OCT analysis demonstrating a thinning area in corneal periphery, allowing direct comparison between scans. (B) An evaluation from November 2013 and (C) an evaluation from January 2016. Even though there are some minimal changes in the thinning morphology, the length is almost equal, and the corneal Dellen can be considered stable during the last years.

(**Figures** 5 and 6) and measure the corneal scar depth before choosing a surgical procedure [12]. A noninvasive surgical technique, such as lamellar keratoplasty (LK) or phototherapeutic keratectomy (PTK), can be chosen when only the anterior corneal layers have been affected, while in other cases, penetrating keratoplasty (PKP) will be the unique option to restore the normal corneal structure. Corneal AS-OCT device also allows direct measurements and comparison with prior scans (**Figure** 5).

Corneal AS-OCT device allows direct measurements and comparison with prior scans (**Figure** 7). The device is essential to evaluate cases with high risk of corneal perforation [13].

Degeneration can be defined as a gradual disruption of the normal condition of a tissue with a subsequent loss of functionality [14]. Corneal degeneration can be related with systemic diseases, local inflammation, or direct toxic action. In this chapter three corneal degenerations will be described: **Salzmann's nodular degeneration (SND), Terrien's marginal degeneration (TMD), and band keratopathy (BK). Arcus senilis** is not present in the developing due to benignant nature of the disease.

2. Salzmann's nodular degeneration

SND is a noninflammatory, slowly progressive, degenerative corneal disease. It is characterized by the presence of elevated, bluish white to gray subepithelial nodules located in the anterior cornea. The size of the nodules oscillates from 1 to 2 mm. Nevertheless, larger nodules have been described as a result of the fusion of several smaller nodules [15, 16] (**Figure 8**).

SND was identified by Maximilian Salzmann in 1925. He described the corneal nodules, usually related to phlyctenular or atheromatous keratitis [17]. SND is often associated with chronic corneal inflammation and irritation. Multiple risk factors have been reported. Interstitial keratitis, vernal keratoconjunctivitis, dry eye disease, meibomian gland dysfunction, pterygium, soft contact lens wearers, and previous trauma or surgical procedures are some disorders that predispose to suffer the pathology.

SND usually occurs in female patients, ranging from 50 to 60 years old. Patients can present unilateral o bilateral disease (**Figure 8**). The number of nodules oscillates from one to eight. These nodules generally adopt a round shape. However, in some cases, they can be conical, prismatic, or wedge-like. Most nodules are avascular although some can be associated with blood vessels. They are normally located in the superior and inferior cornea. In cases of previous pterygium surgery, they will be often located in the edge of the blood vessels; in patients with history of contact lens wearing, in the interpalpebral portion; and in keratoconus patients, in the apex of the cornea.

Corneal AS-OCT SND images display prominent, hyper-reflective, subepithelial deposits overlying Bowman's membrane [1]. The corneal opacities are located under a normally reflective, thin epithelium [10, 16]. The intraepithelial fibrosis overgrowth can result in a corneal surface elevation above Bowman's layer. The central part of nodule has heterogeneous signal intensities, and the nodule margin can be differentiated by subepithelial triangle spike. An irregular stromal scarring can be seen below the nodules, limited to the stromal superficial layers. An epithelial hypertrophy may also be observed around the nodules in an attempt to regularize the corneal surface. The structure of the posterior stroma, Descemet's membrane, and endothelium is not affected by the fibrosis, but the AS-OCT imaging shows a modification of the posterior corneal curvature (**Figure 9**). Both modifications of anterior and posterior corneal curvature induce astigmatic changes and visual loss in these patients.

The destruction of Bowman's layer is considered the most important property in the pathophysiology of the disease [18]. Bowman's layer is replaced by a granular periodic acid Schiff-positive (PAS-positive) eosinophilic material that resembles

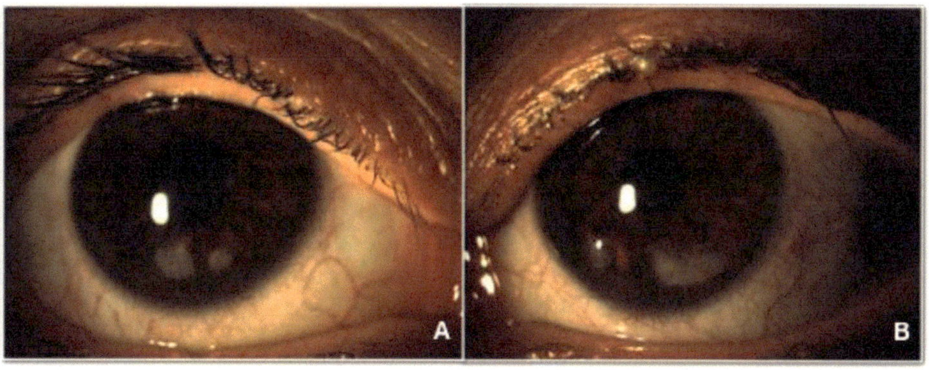

Figure 8.
(A and B) AS slit-lamp biomicroscopy image shows the bluish to white nodules localized in the mid-peripheral inferior cornea. The corneal opacity is present in both eyes of a 56-year-old female SND patient.

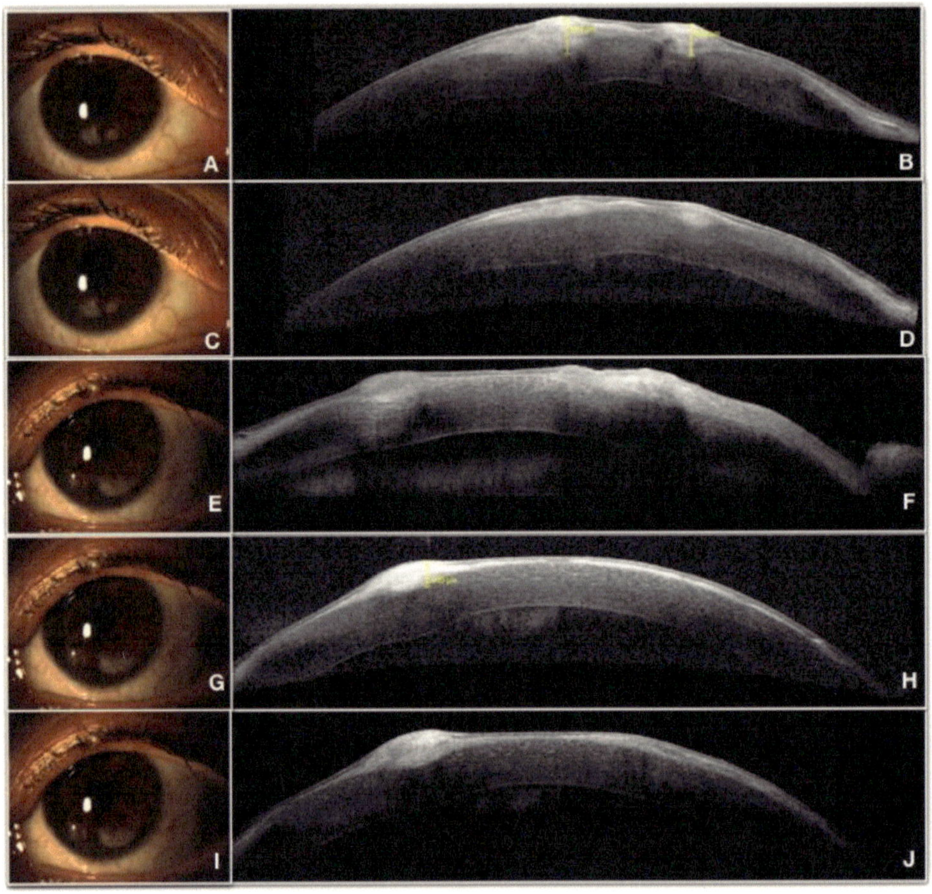

Figure 9.
(A and C) AS slit-lamp biomicroscopy shows two nodules in the right eye of a female patient. (F, H, J) AS-OCT corneal scans display how the prominent nodules overgrow and produce a corneal anterior. (B and D) Corneal AS-OCT images demonstrate the SND nodules localized in the anterior corneal layers, destroying Bowman's layer and producing fibrosis in the anterior stroma. The nodules can be measured using the OCT caliper tool. The device allows the comparison of the nodules sizes between visits. (E, G, I) AS slit-lamp biomicroscopy demonstrates two nodules in the inferior corneal zone on the left eye of the same SND female patient. AS-OCT corneal scans display how the prominent nodules overgrow and produce a corneal anterior surface elevation. The corneal nodules are dense and hyper-reflective. An epithelial hypertrophy may also be observed around the nodules in an attempt to regularize the corneal surface. The structure of the posterior stroma, Descemet's membrane, and endothelium is not affected by the fibrosis, but AS-OCT imaging shows a modification of the posterior corneal curvature.

a basement membrane. The progression of the pathology will be determined by Bowman's layer destruction (**Figure 10**). The involvement of the Bowman layer indicates that surgical delamination of the nodules may be more difficult.

Although most SND cases are asymptomatic, the symptoms can appear depending on the location of the nodules. When they are peripheral, the main symptom is a foreign body sensation, and when they are mid peripheral, the patients complain of decrease in visual acuity. The loss of vision can be attributed to the presence of the corneal opacity and modification of the corneal axis, resulting in an astigmatic change. Other referrals symptoms are severe pain, irritation, and epiphora. The peripheral nodules can produce a flattening of the central cornea, inducing a hyperopic change. This phenomenon has to be considered in the intraocular lens (IOL) power calculation previous to the cataract surgery. The corneal central flattening can cause a refractive postoperative miscalculation [17].

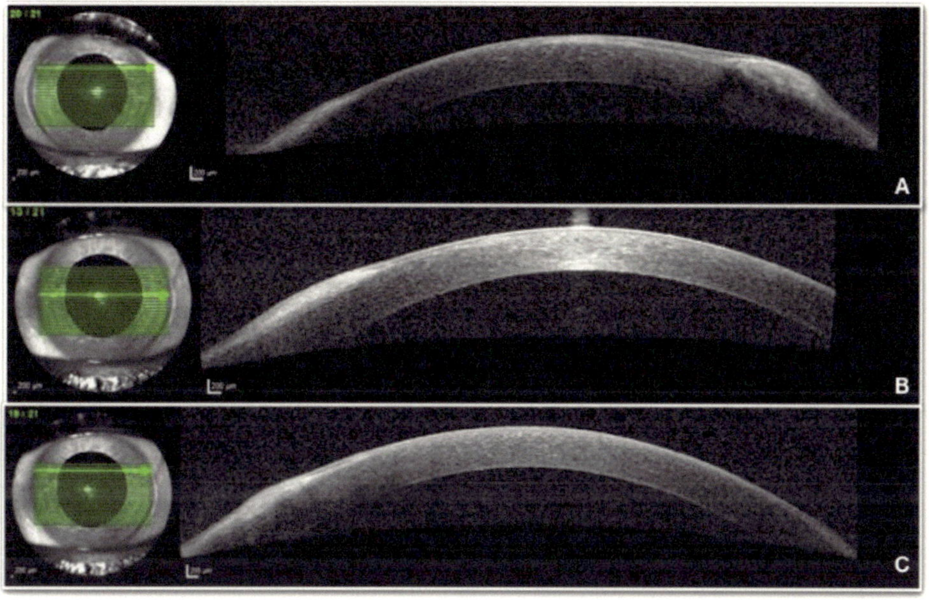

Figure 10.
Corneal AS-OCT evaluation of a SND patient. The scans demonstrate Bowman's layer destruction by the nodule overgrowth. (A) A prominent nodule produces the corneal anterior surface deformation. (B and C) Another nodule extends superficially in the peripheral nasal cornea producing a hyper-reflective area in the subepithelial zone.

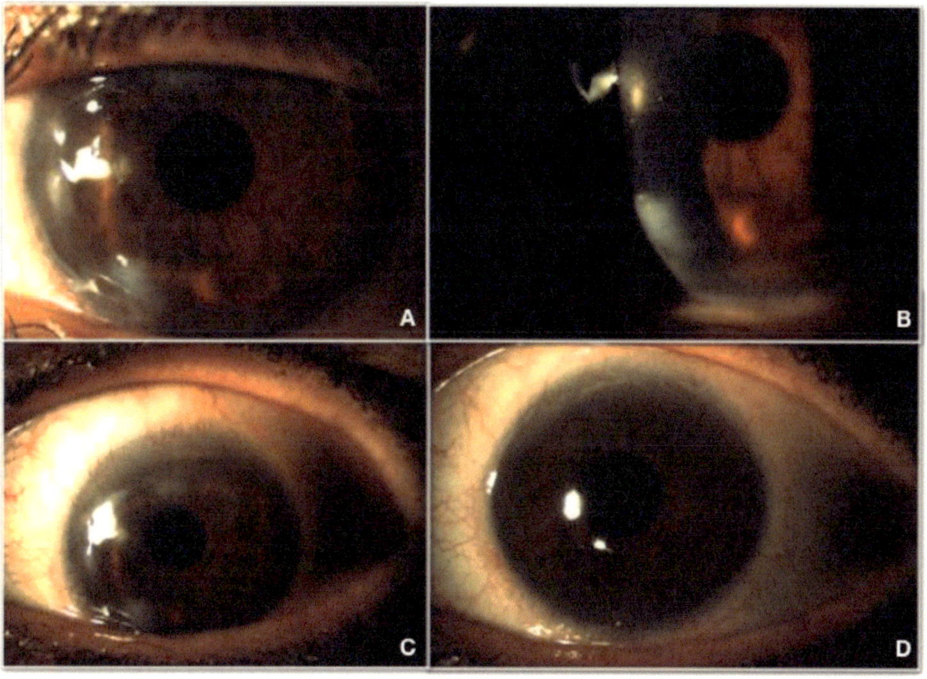

Figure 11.
(A–C) Digital AS slit-lamp biomicroscopy of a SND female patient. The nodules are present all around the peripheral cornea. (D) The same patient following a superficial keratectomy and alcohol-assisted epithelial delamination. The superficial corneal nodules have disappeared.

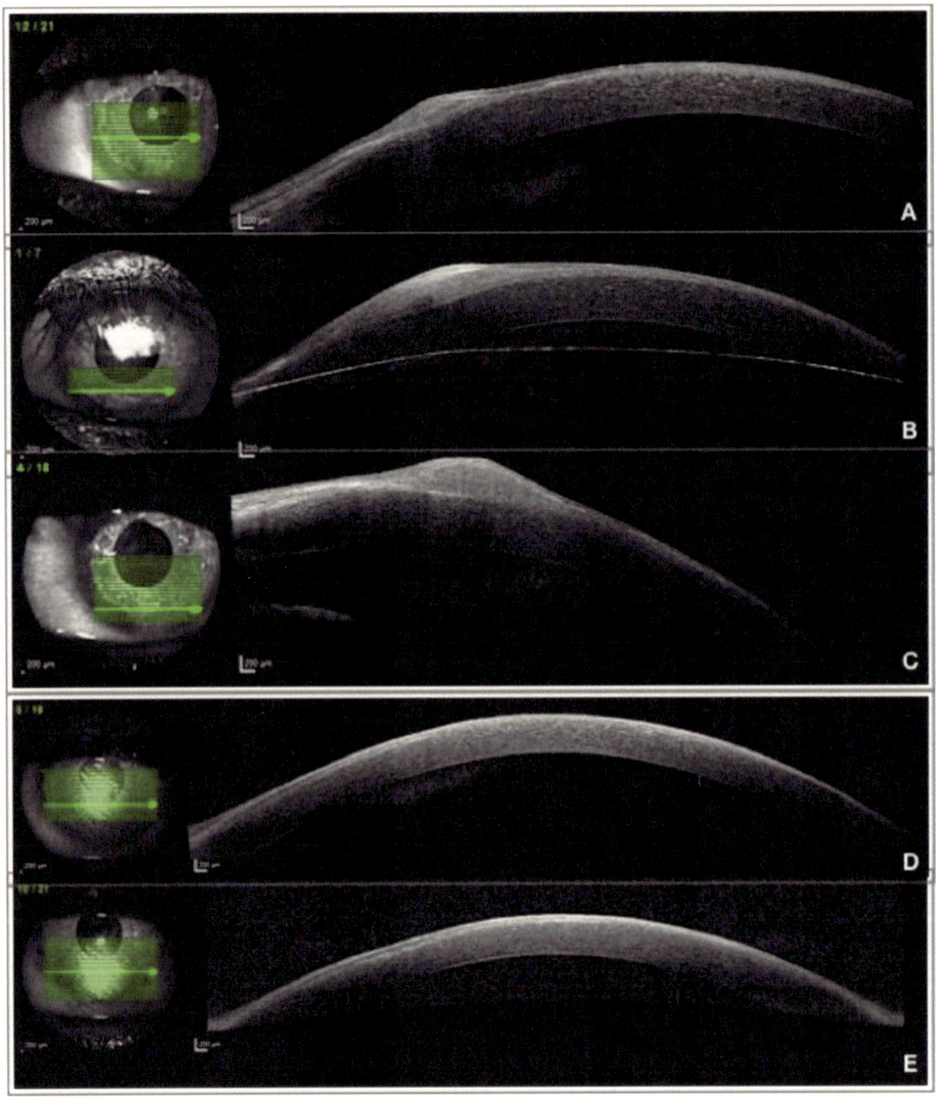

Figure 12.
(A) Corneal AS-OCT analysis of the same SND female patient of ***Figure 11****. (A, B, C) Hyper-reflective nodules can be seen in the mid- peripheral and inferior cornea. (D, E) Corneal AS-OCT scans from the same patient following superficial keratectomy and alcohol-assisted epithelial delamination. The nodules have been removed. The hyper-reflective corneal areas have disappeared, and the anterior surface has restored the morphology.*

In asymptomatic SND patients, conservative treatments will be enough to manage the pathology. The medical therapy with preservative-free lubricants and lid hygiene is appropriated. Autologous serum at 20–50% can be also used. In symptomatic patients, or when inflammation is present, an anti-inflammatory treatment is required. Topical cyclosporine 0.05%, topical preservative-free corticosteroids, and oral doxycycline are useful for the management of SND pathology.

Corneal surgical procedures will be required in persistent symptomatic nodules after medical therapy and in patients with a visual acuity decrease. The main techniques are superficial keratectomy (**Figures 11** and **12**) alone or followed by phototherapeutic keratectomy (PTK). Both procedures can be associated with alcohol-assisted epithelial delamination (**Figures 11** and **12**), amniotic membrane transplantation, or mitomycin-C application.

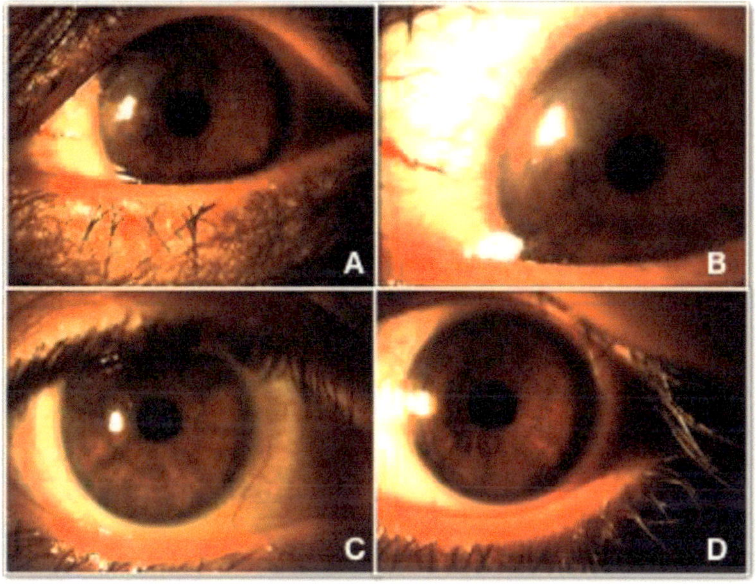

Figure 13.
AS slit-lamp biomicroscopy from a SND patient. (A, B, C) The fibrosis area can be seen in the nasal peripheral corneal zone. (D) The fibrosis has been removed by keratectomy and alcohol-assisted epithelial delamination technique.

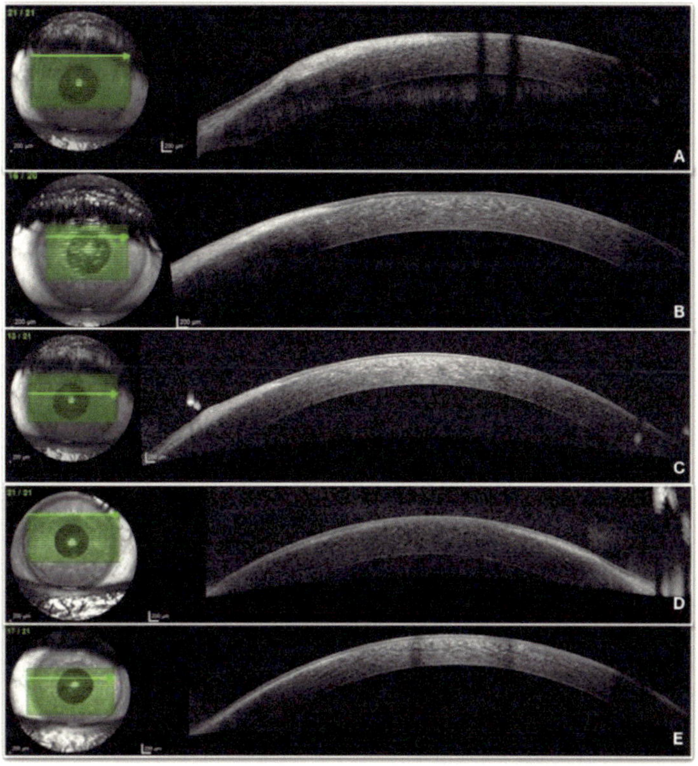

Figure 14.
AS-OCT evaluation from the same SND patient of **Figure 13***. (A–C) The AS-OCT scans show a hyper-reflective zone in the fibrotic areas. (D and E) The fibrosis has been removed by keratectomy and alcohol-assisted epithelial delamination. The hyper-reflective areas are not present.*

Superficial keratectomy will be the surgical first-line therapy in most cases (**Figure 13**). The results will be conditioned by the degree of involvement of the superficial cornea and the degree of affection of the Bowman's layer described in the corneal AS-OCT images (**Figure 14**). An unbroken Bowman's layer or an altered Bowman's layer could be predictive of the strength of the adhesion of the nodules to the anterior stroma [16]. The method used to remove mechanically the opacities will be "peeling the nodules," referred in the bibliography as "Salzmann nodulectomy." In areas of excessive thinning, a careful manual dissection will be required [17].

Keratoplasty will be used in the most severe SND cases. Fortunately, as the mid stroma and Descemet membrane are intact in most SND cases, a lamellar keratoplasty (LK) will be enough to eliminate the opacities. Penetrating keratoplasty (PKP) will be rarely required in SND patients. PKP will be reserved for cases of intraoperative perforation during LK or full-thickness corneal alterations in association with another disease [17].

Corneal AS-OCT images in SND patients have an excellent correlation with the histopathologic exam. AS-OCT analysis is a useful technique that sustained SND diagnosis and helped the clinicians to decide the management and follow-up of the disease progression.

3. Terrien's marginal degeneration (TMD)

TMD is a rare corneal degeneration form. The disease is characterized by a non-ulcerative peripheral corneal thinning [19]. It has a slow and chronic progression, bilaterally and asymmetric. TMD etiology still remains unknown [20]. The pathology has been associated with arthritis and meibomian gland dysfunction. TDM is more frequent in middle-aged males but can occur at any age and in females [21].

TMD is a lipid keratopathy [19]. The slit-lamp biomicroscopy evaluation displays lipid depositions at the edge of the peripheral corneal thinning [21, 22] (**Figure 15**). This lipid accumulation produces yellow-white stromal opacities [22] with superficial neovascularization. Histopathological exams demonstrate intracellular and extracellular vacuoles [21] charged with lipids in the corneal stroma. There is stromal fibrillary degeneration with fatty infiltration of collagen fibers [21, 22]. This stroma degradation produces a decrease in the number of lamellas. TMD lesions have an intact corneal epithelium and an altered Bowman's layer. Electron microscopy studies show the corneal basal membrane and the Bowman layer broken and fragmented.

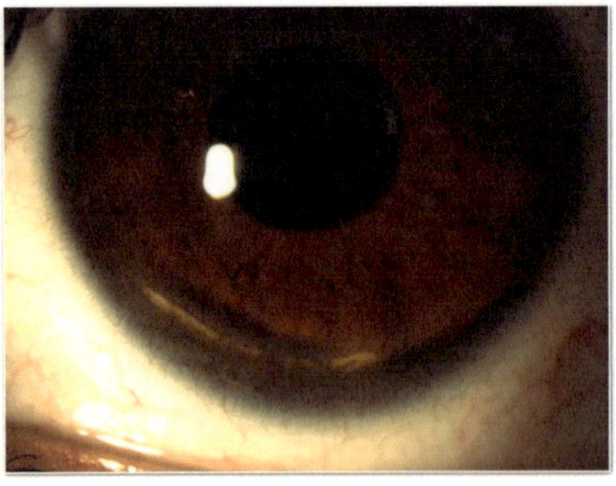

Figure 15.
AS slit-lamp evaluation of a TMD patient. The image demonstrates the lipid deposition in the inferior peripheral corneal area producing yellow-white stromal opacities.

TMD corneal changes can produce an increase in the corneal astigmatism [21], which clinically manifests with a visual acuity decreased. Topography evaluation is essential for a complete pathology study [23].

Two types of TDM have been described. The classic one, more common, generally affects older population [20]. It is usually asymptomatic, noninflammatory, and with a slowly, chronic progress. The second type affects young patients and has a more prominent inflammatory clinical course with a faster evolution [20]. This inflammatory variant is believed to initiate hypersensitivity responses [24, 25] to an immunogenic component of the basal membrane, secreted by the degenerated basal epithelial cells [21]. It can also be produced by phagocytosis of the stromal collagen by histiocyte-like cells [26]. Thinning of the peripheral cornea, corneal opacification, neovascularization, and possible positive fluorescein staining are typically signs of the TMD inflammatory type [21].

Due to the slow progression [22], TMD is generally asymptomatic. Sometimes the diagnosis is incidental because of mild irritation symptoms. Topographic evaluation demonstrates a flattening over the corneal peripheral thinning areas and steepening of the corneal meridian perpendicular to the corneal lesion [21]. TDM slit-lamp biomicroscopy shows the yellowish-white opacities and thinning of the peripheral cornea. The pathology generally initiates at the superior or supero-nasal area. The corneal perforation rate is 15% [21]. It can debut with redness, watering, and sudden decrease of visual acuity. The corneal perforation can cause a deep impact on the vision prognosis regardless of the surgical intervention.

Corneal AS-OCT provides a high-resolution cross-sectional image in TMD patients, and its caliper can take precise and repeatable pachymetry measurements to verify the corneal thickness in the thinner areas (**Figure 16**). It is a safe, rapid, and noninvasive digital technique that depicted structural or morphologic corneal changes. It is a digital precise method to compare the size lesions between the clinical appointments [19, 22]. Medical visits are recommended every 3 months when the minimal corneal thickness is 250 μm [21].

AS-OCT displays the corneal stromal thinning area in TMD disease. The lesions have a non-affected epithelium. In the classic TDM type, the stroma has the same reflectivity as the normal cornea [4]. In the inflammatory TDM, the progressive stromal thinning induces corneal cavity formation with intact epithelial and endothelial layers around the lesion [4, 22] (**Figures 17** and **18**). The external epithelial layer has a normal reflectivity, and the internal endothelial layer is continuous with

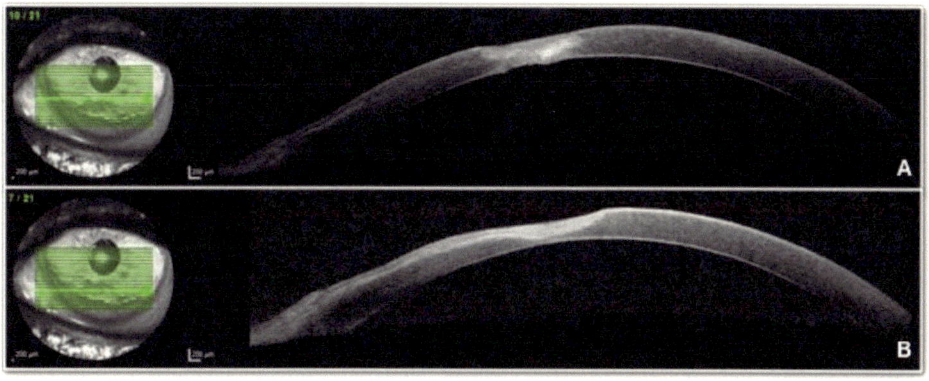

Figure 16.
(A and B) AS-OCT scan demonstrates a corneal thinning area and a hyper-reflective zone in an inflammatory TMD patient. The anterior and the posterior corneal surfaces have their curvatures altered.

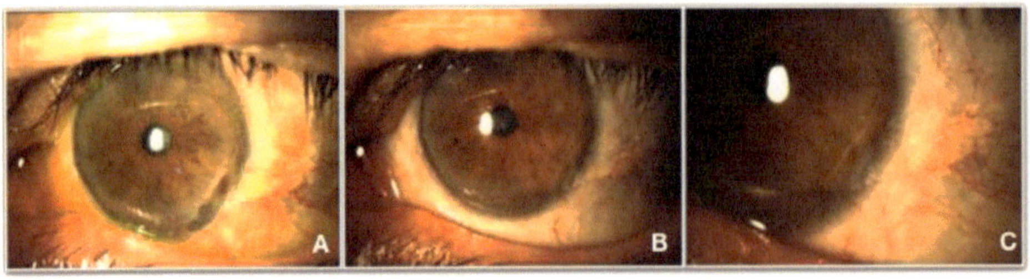

Figure 17.
AS slit-lamp evaluation of a TMD patient. (A) The corneal periphery has a lipid deposition and an extensive thinning area. (B and C) Same TMD patient after an amniotic membrane grafting technique. The image demonstrates how the corneal disorder has been restored.

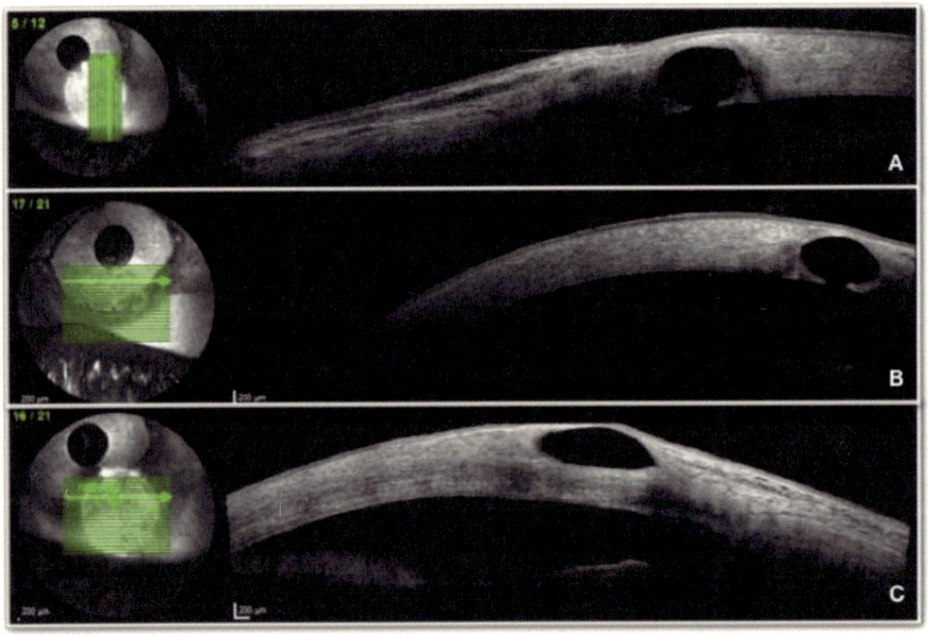

Figure 18.
Corneal AS-OCT of the same TMD patient of ***Figure 17****. (A) Longitudinal scan analysis demonstrates corneal cavitation. (B, C) Transversal scan evaluation also shows the cavitation in the stromal area.*

the rest of the normal endothelial corneal tissue. The corneal thinning areas can show hyper-reflectivity, and AS-OCT evaluation is able to demonstrate corneal cavities not visible in the slit-lamp biomicroscopy [22] (**Figures 17** and **18**).

AS-OCT also evaluates the anterior and the posterior corneal curvatures. Classically, TMD is classified in five clinical stages depending on the disease progression. Recently, a new staging method has been reported [19]. The new classification is based on the anterior and posterior curvatures and the size of the thinnest area, analyzed by corneal AS-OCT. This new staging is useful to evaluate the TMD progression and to plan the surgical management, evidencing the importance of the AS-OCT images to supervise the pathology development.

Due to the slow progression of most TMD cases, the pathology can be managed conservatively in most patients. Noneffective pharmacotherapy has been demonstrated. Nonsurgical interventions include spectacle prescription, rigid gas-permeable contact lenses, scleral lenses, and prosthetic replacement of the ocular surface ecosystem (PROSE) [21]. Eye rubbing has to be avoided.

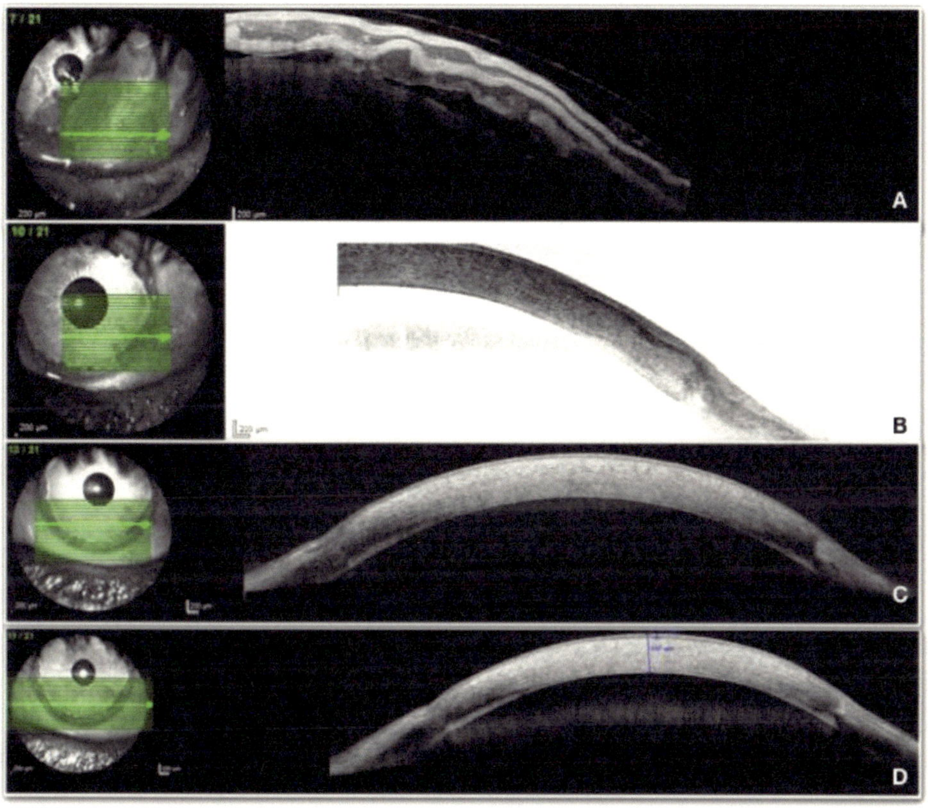

Figure 19.
AS-OCT image from the same TMD patient from ***Figure 18****. (A) The cavitation zone following an amniotic membrane grafting replace technique. The amniotic membrane layers can be distinguished in the scan. (B–D) The image shows how the amniotic membrane has been integrated in the corneal area and has replaced the cavitation zone.*

Surgical procedures are considered when the corneal thickness decreased 150 μm. Nevertheless, some authors prefer an expectant attitude even when the cornea reaches this cross-sectional length [27]. Surgical interventions include the tectonic grafting, whose purpose is to prevent or repair perforation areas in the absence of the donor cornea. The main techniques are conjunctival flaps, scleral autotransplantation, and amniotic membrane grafting (**Figure 19**). Keratoplasty is considered in patients who want to improve their visual acuity. LK is the first technique to consider in this TMD patient [22]. If not, PKP is another possible surgical procedure in more severe cases.

Corneal collagen cross-linking has recently been reported as a good option before performing surgical procedures. It seems to stop the disease evolution, return the thinning area, and improve visual acuity [28].

4. Band keratopathy

Band keratopathy is characterized by calcium deposition in Bowman's layer, most frequently in the interpalpebral zone. The pathology is usually associated with systemic disorders, such as hypercalcemia, or ocular diseases, such as uveitis, chemical burns, intraocular silicone oil, and phthisis eyes after surgeries [28].

AS-OCT imaging is useful for the analysis and measure of the calcium deposition and helpful in achieving a correct pathology management. It shows a

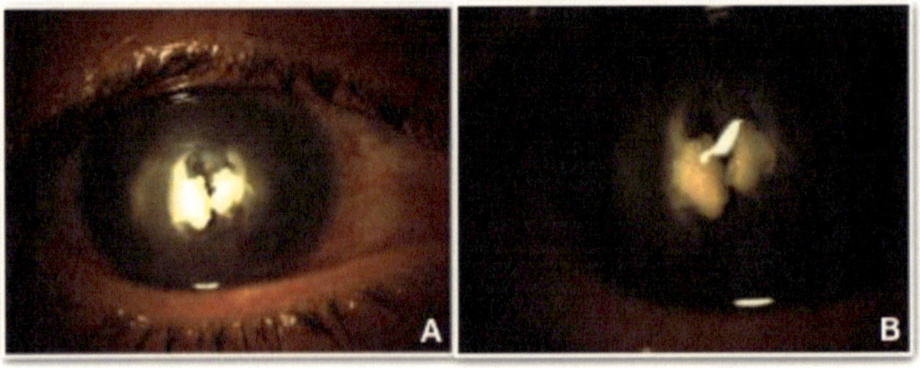

Figure 20.
(A, B) AS slit-lamp evaluation showing calcium deposition in the superficial cornea of a patient with band keratopathy.

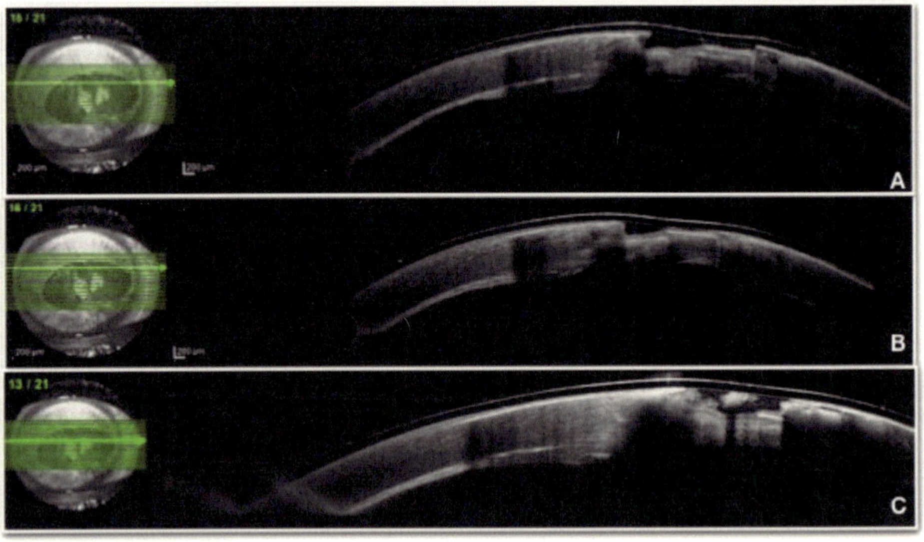

Figure 21.
*(A, B, C) AS-OCT evaluation from the same patient of **Figure 20**. There is a hyper-reflective zone in the calcium deposition areas causing shadows in the corneal stroma below the lesions.*

hyper-reflective material around Bowman's layer causing shadowing in the posterior cornea stroma [3, 29, 30] (**Figures 20** and **21**).

The calcium deposition can result in a loss of visual acuity. The aim of the surgical techniques will be to restore the corneal transparency. AS-OCT imaging can help to decide the optimal surgical technique as the scans show the depth of the lesions [28].

5. Conclusions

AS-OCT imaging is a useful technique that helps physicians to achieve a correct diagnosis and a proper management of the corneal pathologies. Probably, it will become an essential device in the anterior segment disease assessment, as it has occurred in the posterior segment. It is necessary to recognize the AS-OCT specific optical signs of the corneal degenerations, to decide the best therapeutic choice. The scans have to be studied carefully in association with the traditional clinic evaluations. The anterior segment specialists have the responsibility to deepen in the AS-OCT corneal degeneration signs to facilitate the diagnosis and to advance in the knowledge of these pathologies.

Author details

Constanza Caramello Álvarez[1,2]*, María A. del Buey[1,2], Paula Casas[1,2], Sara Marco[1,2], Enrique Mínguez[1,2] and Francisco J. Ascaso[1,2]

1 Department of Ophthalmology, Hospital Clínico Universitario "Lozano Blesa", Zaragoza, Spain

2 Aragon Health Research Institute (IIS Aragon), Zaragoza, Spain

*Address all correspondence to: coni_86@hotmail.com

References

[1] Han SB, Liu YC, Noriega KM, Mehta JS. Applications of anterior segment optical coherence tomography in cornea and ocular surface diseases. Journal of Ophthalmology. 2016;**2016**:4971572

[2] Kanellopoulos AJ, Asimellis G. Anterior-segment optical coherence tomography investigation of corneal deturgescence and epithelial remodeling after DSAEK. Cornea. 2014;**33**:340-348. DOI: 10.1097/ico.0000000000000053

[3] Venkateswaran N. Optical coherence tomography for ocular surface and corneal diseases: A review. Eye and Visión. 2018;**5**:13. DOI: 10.1186/s40662-018-0107-0

[4] Rodriguez M, Yesilirmak N, Chhadva P, Goldhagen B, Karp C, Galor A. High-resolution optical coherence tomography in the differentiation of inflammatory versus noninflammatory peripheral corneal thinning. Cornea. 2017;**36**:48-52

[5] Yasuno Y, Madjarova VD, Makita S, Akiba M, Morosawa A, Chong C, et al. Three-dimensional and high-speed swept-source optical coherence tomography for in vivo investigation of human anterior eye segments. Optics Express. 2005;**13**:10652-10664

[6] Shapiro BL, Cortés DE, Chin EK, et al. High-resolution spectral domain anterior segment optical coherence tomography in type 1 Boston keratoprosthesis. Cornea. 2013;**32**:951-955

[7] Vajzovic LM, Karp CL, Haft P, Shousha MA, Dubovy SR, Hurmeric V, et al. Ultra high-resolution anterior segment optical coherence tomography in the evaluation of anterior corneal dystrophies and degenerations. Ophthalmology. 2011;**118**:1291-1296. DOI: 10.1016/j.ophtha.2010.12.015

[8] Kieval JZ, Karp CL, Abou Shousha M, Galor A, Hoffman RA, Dubovy SR, et al. Ultra-high resolution optical coherence tomography for differentiation of ocular surface squamous neoplasia and pterygia. Ophthalmology. 2012;**119**:481-486. DOI: 10.1016/j.ophtha.2011.08.028

[9] Thomas BJ, Galor A, Nanji AA, El Sayyad F, Wang J, Dubovy SR, et al. Ultra high-resolution anterior segment optical coherence tomography in the diagnosis and management of ocular surface squamous neoplasia. The Ocular Surface. 2014;**12**:46-58. DOI: 10.1016/j.jtos.2013.11.001

[10] Nanji AA, Sayyad FE, Galor A, Dubovy S, Karp CL. High-resolution optical coherence tomography as an adjunctive tool in the diagnosis of corneal and conjunctival pathology. The Ocular Surface. 2015;**13**:226-235. DOI: 10.1016/j.jtos.2015.02.001

[11] Shousha MA, Karp CL, Canto AP, Hodson K, Oellers P, Kao AA, et al. Diagnosis of ocular surface lesions using ultra-high-resolution optical coherence tomography. Ophthalmology. 2013;**120**:883-891. DOI: 10.1016/j.ophtha.2012.10.025

[12] Zhou SY, Wang CX, Cai XY, Huang D, Liu YZ. Optical coherence tomography and ultrasound biomicroscopy imaging of opaque corneas. Cornea. 2013;**32**:e25-e30

[13] Ang M, Baskaran M, Werkmeister RM, Chua J, Schmidl D, Aranha Dos Santos V, et al. Anterior segment optical coherence tomography. Progress in Retinal and Eye Research. 2018;**66**:132-156. DOI: 10.1016/j.preteyeres.2018.04.002

[14] Trufanov SV, Salovarova EP, Tekeeva LY. Corneal degenerations. Vestnik Oftalmologii. 2018;**134**:282-288. DOI: 10.17116/oftalma2018134051282

[15] Marcon AS, Rapuano CJ. Excimer laser phototherapeutic keratectomy retreatment of anterior basement membrane dystrophy and Salzmann's nodular degeneration with topical mitomycin C. Cornea. 2002;**21**:828-830

[16] Hurmeric V, Yoo SH, Karp CL, et al. In vivo morphologic characteristics of Salzmann nodular degeneration with ultra-high-resolution optical coherence tomography. American Journal of Ophthalmology. 2010;**151**:248-256.e2

[17] Maharana PK, Sharma N, Das S, Agarwal T, Sen S, Prakash G, et al. Salzmann's nodular degeneration. The Ocular Surface. 2016;**14**:20-30. DOI: 10.1016/j.jtos.2015.08.006

[18] Das S, Link B, Seitz B. Salzmann's nodular degeneration of the cornea: A review and case series. Cornea. 2005;**24**:772-777

[19] Wang N, Wang CX, Lian XF, Duan SJ, Huang D, Zhou SY. Staging of development in Terrien's degeneration based on corneal curvatures detected by optical coherence tomography. Graefe's Archive for Clinical and Experimental Ophthalmology. 2015;**253**:1757-1764. DOI: 10.1007/s00417-015-3057-4

[20] Lee TL, Lee HY, Tan JCH. Terrien marginal degeneration complicated by a corneoscleral cyst. Cornea. 2018;**37**:658-660. DOI: 10.1097/ICO.0000000000001546

[21] Ding Y, Murri MS, Birdsong OC, Ronquillo Y, Moshirfar M. Terrien marginal degeneration. Survey of Ophthalmology. 12 Oct 2018. pii: S0039-6257(18)30047-X. DOI: 10.1016/j.survophthal.2018.09.004. Review. PubMed PMID: 30316804. [Epub ahead of print]

[22] Hattori T, Kumakura S, Mori H, Goto H. Depiction of cavity formation in Terrien marginal degeneration by anterior segment optical coherence tomography. Cornea. 2013;**32**:615-618. DOI: 10.1097/ICO.0b013e318259c970

[23] Fernandes M. Scanning slit topography: Diagnostic boon in presumed unilateral Terrien's marginal degeneration. Contact Lens & Anterior Eye. 2011;**34**:282-286

[24] Iwamoto T, DeVoe a FRL. Electron microscopy in cases of marginal degeneration of the cornea. Investigative Ophthalmology. 1972;**11**:241-257

[25] Austin P, Brown SI. Inflammatory Terrien's marginal corneal disease. American Journal of Ophthalmology. 1981;**92**:189-192

[26] Süveges I, Lévai G, Alberth B. Pathology of Terrien's disease: Histochemical and electron microscopic study. American Journal of Ophthalmology. 1972;**74**:1191-1200. DOI: 10.1016/0002-9394(72)90742-8

[27] Galvis V, Tello A, Niño CA, Larrea J. Terrien marginal degeneration: Clinical characteristics and outcomes. American Journal of Ophthalmology. 2016;**164**:151-152. DOI: 10.1016/j.ajo.2016.01.001

[28] Hafezi F, Gatzioufas Z, Seiler TG, Seiler T. Corneal collagen cross-linking for Terrien marginal degeneration. Journal of Refractive Surgery. 2014;**30**:498-500. DOI: 10.3928/1081597X-20140527-02

[29] Mansour AM, Haddad R. Optical coherence tomography of band keratopathy. BML Case Reports. 2016;**2016**: pii: bcr2016218216. doi: 10.1136/bcr-2016-218216

[30] Moisseiev E, Gal A, Addadi L, Caspi D, Shemesh G, Michaeli A. Acute calcific band keratopathy: Case report and literature review. Journal of Cataract and Refractive Surgery. 2013;**39**:292-294. DOI: 10.1016/j.jcrs.2012.12.020

Chapter 3

Intraoperative OCT for Monitoring Corneal Pachymetry during Corneal Collagen Cross-Linking for Keratoconus

Reza Ghaffari, Hassan Hashemi and Soheila Asghari

Abstract

Biomechanical reinforcement of the cornea by collagen cross-linking (CXL) using riboflavin and ultraviolet A (UV-A) irradiation is a well-established treatment for halting the progression of keratoconus. Corneal pachymetry is one of the most important factors with respect to the safety of CXL. In addition to the initial pachymetric changes, significant changes in corneal pachymetry may occur during the different steps of the procedure, highlighting the role of intraoperative pachymetric measurements. Intraoperative optical coherence tomography (OCT) can be used safely and effectively to monitor the corneal pachymetry during CXL. Among the advantages of this technology is its ability to provide a more detailed profile of the corneal thickness in a noncontact manner compared to the ultrasound method. These features are especially advantageous for monitoring corneal pachymetry in the setting of CXL in KCN patients, considering the marked irregularity of the epithelium and stroma in these patients. OCT has also been used for evaluation of other aspects of the CXL procedure like evaluation of in vivo riboflavin penetration in to the corneal stroma.

Keywords: anterior segment OCT, keratoconus, collagen cross-linking, intraoperative OCT, corneal pachymetry

1. Introduction

Keratoconus is a bilateral, progressive, ectatic disease characterized by progressive corneal thinning and irregular astigmatism. Biomechanical instability of the cornea is considered a main feature contributing to disease manifestations and a hallmark of this disease [1].

Biomechanical reinforcement of the cornea by collagen cross-linking (CXL) using riboflavin as a photosensitizer and ultraviolet A (UV-A) irradiation is a well-established treatment for halting the progression of keratoconus [2, 3].

The CXL process is mediated by a photo-oxidation reaction between UV-A (370 nm) and riboflavin (vitamin B2). Reactive oxygen species produced during this reaction, including singlet oxygen, react with the collagen fibril molecules in corneal stroma and enhance the mechanical strength of cornea by forming new chemical bonds between collagen fibril molecules [4].

The original procedure (Dresden protocol) includes removal of the central 7 mm of the corneal epithelium (epithelium-off method), riboflavin saturation of the stroma with 0.1% riboflavin-20% dextran solution (every 5 minutes until 30 minutes), and then application of UV-A light source (370 nm with irradiance of 3 mW/cm^2) on the cornea for 30 minutes [2]. However, there have been other modifications such as preserving the corneal epithelium (epithelial-on method), increasing the intensity of the UV source and decreasing the irradiation time (accelerated method), and using a continuous versus a pulsed light source after the description of the original procedure.

A significant increase up to 71.9 and 328.9% in corneal rigidity has been demonstrated in experimental studies in porcine and human corneas, respectively [4], and long-term studies have demonstrated the safety and efficacy of CXL in halting the progression of keratoconus [5, 6].

2. Significance of corneal pachymetry as a safety criteria for CXL

Corneal thickness (measured by pachymetry) is one of the most important factors with respect to the safety of CXL; a minimum thickness of 400 μm is recommended to ensure the safety of the procedure and avoid the potential toxic effects of UV-A irradiation on the corneal endothelium [7]. Both an adequate corneal thickness and adequate riboflavin saturation of the cornea are necessary to ensure photochemical damage caused by the free radicals to the corneal endothelium.

With the currently used irradiation doses in CXL (UV-A radiant exposure of 5.4 mJ/cm^2 and the corresponding irradiance of 3 mW/cm^2), the estimated level of irradiance at a depth of 400 μm is 0.18 mW/cm^2 which is by two factors below the damage threshold [7].

CXL in thin corneas with a minimum corneal thickness below 400 μm after epithelial removal has been reported to result in significant endothelial cell loss postoperatively, emphasizing the role of corneal pachymetry as a critical factor for the CXL procedure [8].

3. Pachymetric changes during CXL for KCN and importance of intraoperative pachymetric monitoring

In addition to the initial pachymetric changes, significant changes in corneal pachymetry may occur during the different steps of the procedure [9–11]. Factors contributing to these changes include epithelial removal, dehydration due to corneal stroma due to exposure, osmotic effects of the riboflavin-dextran solution, and UV irradiation. The use of an eyelid speculum during instillation of riboflavin drops and the dextran containing riboflavin formulations (as compared to non-dextran containing riboflavin iso-osmolar formulations) are especially among the potential factors associated with shrinkage of the corneal stroma during the procedure.

Kymionis et al. [10] reported a decrease of 75 μm and Muzzotta et al. [11] reported a 32.07% shrinkage of the corneal stromal thickness after riboflavin saturation of the stroma with the riboflavin-dextran solution. These findings indicate that despite an initial pachymetry value greater than 400 μm, a considerable proportion of patients will end up with a corneal pachymetry value below the critical thickness during the procedure, which may be a factor explaining complications like corneal edema despite an initial adequate pachymetry in some reports [12].

These pachymetric changes all could potentially jeopardize the safety of the procedure, further highlighting the importance of intraoperative pachymetric monitoring during the operation.

DOI: http://dx.doi.org/10.5772/intechopen.84243

4. Current standard method used for intraoperative corneal pachymetry measurements

Currently, ultrasound pachymetry is the most commonly used method for intraoperative pachymetry measurements during CXL. However, pachymetry measurements using this technique are subject to limitations: only single point measurements can be obtained and it is necessary to have contact to obtain the measurements, thus making the results more prone to inter- and intra-observer variability. In addition, vulnerability to infections due to contact with the surface of the eye and inadequate sterilization of the ultrasound tip during the procedure is another concern associated with this method.

5. Application of intraoperative OCT for corneal pachymetry during collagen cross-linking

5.1 Advantages of OCT as a diagnostic tool for corneal imaging

Anterior segment optical coherence tomography (AS-OCT) is a noninvasive imaging modality that can be used to obtain high-resolution, cross-sectional images of the anterior structures of the eye. In comparison with ultrasound pachymetry, AS-OCT has the advantage of providing a more detailed corneal anatomic profile during the procedure with a high degree of intra-observer repeatability and inter-observer reproducibility of the pachymetric measurements.

OCT has been proven to be a useful diagnostic imaging modality for the diagnosis of keratoconus. OCT-derived corneal thickness distribution and asymmetry parameters have been shown to have a good correlation with established Scheimpflug-derived anterior surface irregularity indices and proven useful to detect suspect, early, and clinical keratoconus [13].

The high resolution of the spectral domain OCT which allows for reconstruction of epithelial and stromal thickness profiles is another advantage of OCT to study the altered epithelial thickness pattern in keratoconus due to corneal surface irregularity. OCT-derived epithelial thickness map parameters have shown promising results in early and advanced keratoconus detection [14, 15].

OCT has also been used for detection of demarcation lines after CXL which are considered as a measure of the treatment efficacy [16]. In addition, OCT has been proved to be useful to show changes after CXL including the epithelial remodeling after CXL, resulting in a thinner and more regular thickness profile [7].

5.2 Application of intraoperative OCT in corneal and anterior segment surgery

OCT as a real-time and high-resolution imaging modality provides additional information regarding the angle, corneal thickness, and other structures that are otherwise invisible or difficult to visualize using the normal operating microscope, making it a potential beneficial tool for anterior segment surgery. In addition, it could provide valuable information in the cases like corneal opacity which preclude visualization of the anterior segment structures of the eye.

Intraoperative OCT has also been used as a useful extension of the normal surgical microscope during anterior segment procedures for finding the plane of corneal dissection during anterior lamellar surgery, for assessment of graft-host relationship in penetrating keratoplasty, as a guide during the crucial aspects of posterior lamellar surgery, cataract surgery, and glaucoma procedures like canaloplasty or trabectome surgery [17–22].

As another application of intraoperative OCT, this modality has been used for anterior segment examination of patients under general anesthesia, diagnosis of complex wound apposition problems, with the advantage of providing additional information for understanding corneal wound-related problems [23].

With the adaptation of this technology, intraoperative online OCT provides additional information for anterior segment surgeons providing a real-time dynamic feedback of the various surgical steps during surgery. Nonetheless, shadowing produced by surgical instruments represents the main limitation of this technology [19].

5.3 Application of intraoperative OCT for monitoring corneal pachymetry during corneal collagen cross-linking

Intraoperative OCT has been used to monitor the corneal pachymetry during CXL. The high resolution of OCT is especially advantageous in KCN patients, considering the marked epithelial and stromal irregularity in these patients.

In a study, Mazzotta and Karagiuli reported corneal pachymetric measurements in patients with keratoconus undergoing CXL. Pachymetric measurements were performed before, during, and after instillation of riboflavin using the time-domain Visante OCT (Zeiss, Jena, Germany). They showed significant corneal stromal shrinkage during the instillation of the riboflavin 0.1%-dextran T500 20% solution with 17.61, 25.44, and 32.07% reduction in the corneal thickness after 10, 20, and 30 minutes of riboflavin instillation, respectively [9].

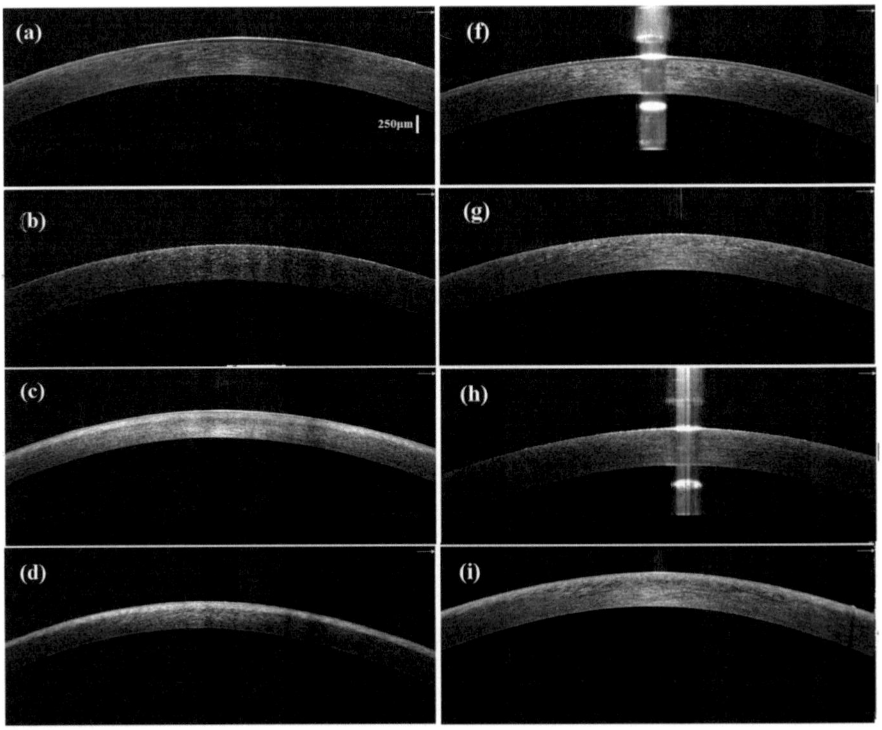

Figure 1.
Representative intraoperative OCT images of cases in the speculum-on (a–d) and speculum-off (f–i) groups. The images represent different stages of the procedure: at the baseline (a, f), after epithelial removal (b, g), after riboflavin saturation of the corneal stroma (c, h), and after UV-A irradiation (d, i).

In another study, Rechichi et al. used intraoperative OCT to evaluate corneal pachymetry in keratoconic patients undergoing accelerated corneal collagen cross-linking with a dextran-free 0.1% riboflavin solution plus hydroxyl-propyl methylcellulose (HPMC). Intraoperative corneal thickness was evaluated by corneal optical coherence tomography (iVUE Optovue Inc., Fremont, CA, USA). Their results showed a central corneal thickness of 388.5 ± 36.8, 385.2 ± 37.8, and 379.4 ± 37.2 μm after epithelial removal, after 10 minutes of soaking with riboflavin, and after ultraviolet instillation, respectively. Their findings are compatible with those of a stable corneal pachymetry with the dextran-free riboflavin solution, throughout the procedure [24].

In our study, we used intraoperative OCT to compare the effect of eyelid speculum on corneal pachymetric changes using an accelerated (9 mW/cm^2 for 10 minutes) CXL protocol. In 14 patients, the speculum was removed during the riboflavin imbibition time (speculum-off group), while in 11 patients the speculum was retained during this period (speculum-on group). Intraoperative OCT (iVue 100-2; Optovue, Fremont, CA, USA) was used to measure the corneal thickness at baseline, after epithelial removal, after 30 minutes of 0.1% riboflavin in 20% dextran T-500 solution instillation, and after irradiation. The speculum-on group showed a significantly greater decrease in the corneal pachymetry (83.7 vs. 16.4 μm decrease in corneal thickness) during riboflavin instillation. As shown in the **Figures 1** and **2**, the speculum-off group had a more stable corneal pachymetry value during riboflavin instillation. On the other hand, the speculum-off group had a greater decrease in the corneal pachymetry value during the irradiation phase, further highlighting the limitations imposed by corneal stromal shrinkage using the isotonic dextran containing riboflavin solution for CXL [25].

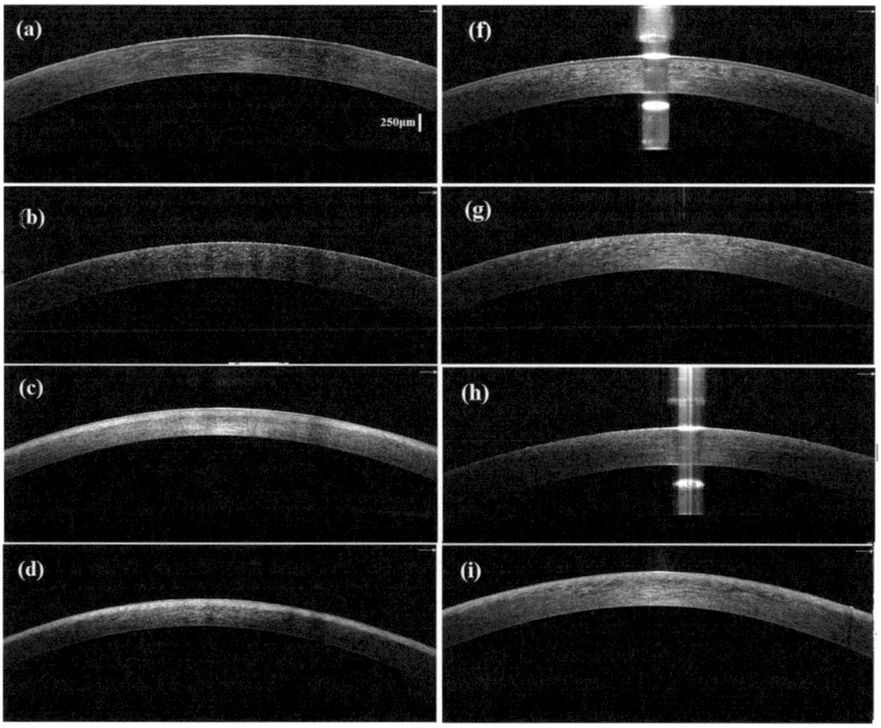

Figure 2.
Representative OCT corneal thickness maps in the speculum-on (a–d) and speculum-off (f–i) groups. Note the marked thinning observed in the corneal thickness map during the riboflavin-dextran instillation of the cornea in the speculum-on group (c, h).

6. Other applications of intraoperative OCT for corneal collagen cross-linking

OCT has been used for in vivo evaluation of the riboflavin penetration to the stroma during CXL.

Riboflavin penetration of the cornea is associated with a hyper-reflective signal change in the corneal stroma. Although the correlation between the band's intensity and riboflavin stromal concentration has not been directly investigated, it is speculated that a higher OCT reflectivity should be positively correlated with riboflavin concentration.

Mahotra et al. evaluated the depth of hyper-reflective band (representing penetration of riboflavin) in the anterior corneal stroma after riboflavin saturation of the stroma in 20 patients undergoing CXL with either complete epithelial removal or grid-like epithelial removal (leaving behind intact islands of epithelium) using hand-held spectral domain OCT. In the complete removal group, the hyper-reflective band was homogenous, extending to a mean depth of 54.2 ± 5.2 µm in the stroma. However, the hyper-reflective band was uneven in the grid pattern epithelial removal [26].

Vinciguerra et al. measured the depth of hyper-reflective band after riboflavin saturation of the stroma using two different methods (epithelium-off and iontophoresis method) in six patients. In the conventional epi-off group, after 30 minutes of riboflavin instillation, a homogeneous hyper-reflective band without fading was measured at a mean depth of 80 µm. In the iontophoresis group, a less homogeneous but deeper hyper-reflective band with a fading effect was observed extending through the anterior 200 µm of the cornea [27].

Pahuja et al. used a microscope-integrated real-time spectral domain optical coherence tomography (ZEISS OPMI LUMERA 700 and ZEISS RESCAN 700) to compare the penetration of riboflavin between epithelium-on and epithelium-off methods in keratoconus patients undergoing accelerated CXL. The mean depth of the hyper-reflective stromal band was 149.39 and 191.04 microns in the epithelium-on and epithelium-off groups, respectively. These results are compatible with enhanced riboflavin corneal penetration with the epithelium-off method [28].

7. Conclusions

Intraoperative OCT can be used safely and effectively to monitor corneal pachymetry during CXL. Among the advantages of this technology is its ability to provide a more detailed profile of the corneal thickness in a noncontact manner, which is especially advantageous for monitoring corneal pachymetry in the setting of CXL in KCN patients compared to the conventional ultrasound method. OCT has also been used for evaluation of other aspects of the CXL procedure like evaluation of in vivo riboflavin penetration in to the corneal stroma.

Conflict of interest

The authors declare no conflict of interest regarding any material related to the article.

Author details

Reza Ghaffari[1]*, Hassan Hashemi[2] and Soheila Asghari[3]

1 Farabi Eye Hospital, Tehran, Iran

2 Noor Research Center for Ophthalmic Epidemiology, Noor Eye Hospital, Tehran, Iran

3 Noor Ophthalmology Research Center, Noor Eye Hospital, Tehran, Iran

*Address all correspondence to: ghaffaryreza@yahoo.com

References

[1] Rabinowitz YS. Keratoconus. Survey of Ophthalmology. 1998;**42**(4):297-319. DOI: 10.1016/S0039-6257(97)00119-7

[2] Wollensak G, Spoerl E, Seiler T. Riboflavin/ultraviolet-a induced collagen crosslinking for the treatment of keratoconus. American Journal of Ophthalmology. 2003;**135**(5):620-627. DOI: 10.1016/S0039-6257(97)00119-7

[3] Wollensak G. Crosslinking treatment of progressive keratoconus: New hope. Current Opinion in Ophthalmology. 2006;**17**(4):356-360. DOI: 10.1097/01.icu.0000233954.86723.25

[4] Wollensak G, Spoerl E, Seiler T. Stress-strain measurements of human and porcine corneas after riboflavin-ultraviolet-A-induced cross-linking. Journal of Cataract and Refractive Surgery. 2003;**29**(9):1780-1785. DOI: 10.1016/S0886-3350(03)00407-3

[5] Theuring A, Spoerl E, Pillunat L, Raiskup F. Corneal collagen cross-linking with riboflavin and ultraviolet-a light in progressive keratoconus: Results after 10-year follow-up. Der Ophthalmologe. 2015;**112**(2):140-147. DOI: 10.1007/s00347-014-3114-0

[6] Hashemi H, Seyedian MA, Miraftab M, Fotouhi A, Asgari S. Corneal collagen cross linking with riboflavin and ultraviolet a irradiation for keratoconus: Long-term results. Ophthalmology. 2013;**120**(8):1515-1520. DOI: 10.1016/j.ophtha.2013.01.012

[7] Spoerl E, Mrochen M, Sliney D, Trokel S, Seiler T. Safety of UVA-riboflavin cross-linking of the cornea. Cornea. 2007;**26**(4):385-389. DOI: 10.1097/ICO.0b013e3180334f78

[8] Kymionis GD, Portaliou DM, Diakonis VF, Kounis GA, Panagopoulou SI, Grentzelos MA. Corneal collagen cross-linking with riboflavin and ultraviolet-a irradiation in patients with thin corneas. American Journal of Ophthalmology. 2012;**153**(1):24-28. DOI: 10.1016/j.ajo.2011.05.036

[9] Mazzotta C, Caragiuli S. Intraoperative corneal thickness measurement by optical coherence tomography in keratoconic patients undergoing corneal collagen cross-linking. American Journal of Ophthalmology. 2014;**157**(6):1156-1162. DOI: 10.1016/j.ajo.2014.02.042

[10] Kymionis GD, Kounis GA, Portaliou DM, Grentzelos MA, Karavitaki AE, Coskunseven E, et al. Intraoperative pachymetric measurements during corneal collagen crosslinking with riboflavin and ultraviolet a irradiation. Ophthalmology. 2009;**116**(12):2336-2339. DOI: 10.1016/j.ophtha.2009.09.018

[11] Schmidinger G, Pachala M, Prager F. Pachymetry changes during corneal crosslinking: Effect of closed eyelids and hypotonic riboflavin solution. Journal of Cataract and Refractive Surgery. 2013;**39**(8):1179-1183. DOI: 10.1016/j.jcrs.2013.03.021

[12] Gokhale NS. Corneal endothelial damage after collagen cross-linking treatment. Cornea. 2011;**30**(12):1495-1498. DOI: 10.1097/ICO.0b013e31820687f7

[13] Kanellopoulos AJ, Asimellis G. OCT-derived comparison of corneal thickness distribution and asymmetry differences between normal and keratoconic eyes. Cornea. 2014;**33**(12):1274-1281. DOI: 10.1097/ICO.0000000000000275

[14] Kanellopoulos AJ, Asimellis G. OCT corneal epithelial topographic asymmetry as a sensitive diagnostic tool for early and advancing keratoconus. Clinical Ophthalmology. 2014;**8**:2277-2287. DOI: 10.2147%2FOPTH.S67902

[15] Li Y, Tan O, Brass R, Weiss JL, Huang D. Corneal epithelial thickness mapping by Fourier-domain optical coherence tomography in normal and keratoconic eyes. Ophthalmology. 2012;**119**(12):2425-2433. DOI: 10.1016/j.ophtha.2012.06.023

[16] Doors M, Tahzib NG, Eggink FA, Berendschot TT, Webers CA, Nuijts RM. Use of anterior segment optical coherence tomography to study corneal changes after collagen cross-linking. American Journal of Ophthalmology. 2009;**148**(6):844-851. DOI: 10.1016/j.ajo.2009.06.031

[17] Atia R, Jouve L, Sandali O, Laroche L, Borderie V, Bouheraoua N. Early epithelial remodeling after standard and Iontophoresis-assisted corneal cross-linking as evaluated by spectral-domain optical coherence tomography. Journal of Refractive Surgery. 2018;**34**(8):551-558. DOI: 10.3928/1081597X-20180702-01

[18] Siebelmann S, Bachmann B, Lappas A, Dietlein T, Steven P, Cursiefen C. Intraoperative optical coherence tomography for examination of newborns and infants under general anesthesia. Der Ophthalmologe. 2016;**113**(8):651-655. DOI: 10.1007/s00347-016-0299-4

[19] Siebelmann S, Bachmann B, Lappas A, Dietlein T, Hermann M, Roters S, et al. Intraoperative optical coherence tomography in corneal and glaucoma surgical procedures. Der Ophthalmologe. 2016;**113**(8):646-650. DOI: 10.1007/s00347-016-0320-y

[20] Wylegala E, Nowinska AK, Wroblewska-Czajka E, Janiszewska D. Donor disc attachment assessment with intraoperative spectral optical coherence tomography during descemet stripping automated endothelial keratoplasty. Indian Journal of Ophthalmology. 2013;**61**(9):511-513. DOI: 10.4103%2F0301-4738.119440

[21] Steven P, Le Blanc C, Velten K, Lankenau E, Krug M, Oelckers S, et al. Optimizing descemet membrane endothelial keratoplasty using intraoperative optical coherence tomography. JAMA Ophthalmology. 2013;**131**(9):1135-1142. DOI: 10.1001/jamaophthalmol.2013.4672

[22] Titiyal J, Kaur M, Falera R. Intraoperative optical coherence tomography in anterior segment surgeries. Indian Journal of Ophthalmology. 2017;**65**:116. DOI: 10.4103%2Fijo.IJO_868_16

[23] Pujari A, Mukhija R, Urkude J, Singh R, Agarwal D, Sharma N. Intraoperative assessment of corneal injuries using microscope-integrated optical coherence tomography. Indian Journal of Ophthalmology. 2018;**66**(11):1614-1615. DOI: 10.4103%2Fijo.IJO_546_18

[24] Rechichi M, Mazzotta C, Daya S, Mencucci R, Lanza M, Meduri A. Intraoperative OCT Pachymetry in patients undergoing dextran-free riboflavin UVA accelerated corneal collagen crosslinking. Current Eye Research. 2016;**41**(10):1310-1315. DOI: 10.3109/02713683.2015.1118130

[25] Ghaffari R, Mortazavi M, Anvari P, Salamat Rad A, Alipour F, Hafezi F, et al. Intraoperative optical coherence tomography to evaluate the effect of the eyelid speculum on corneal pachymetry during accelerated corneal cross-linking (9 mW/cm^2). Eye. 2018;**32**(3):579-585. DOI: 10.1038/eye.2017.243

[26] Malhotra C, Shetty R, Kumar RS, Veluri H, Nagaraj H, Shetty KB. In vivo imaging of riboflavin penetration during collagen cross-linking with hand-held spectral domain optical coherence tomography. Journal of Refractive Surgery. 2012;**28**(11):776-780. DOI: 10.3928/1081597X-20121011-05

[27] Vinciguerra P, Rechichi M, Rosetta P, Romano MR, Mastropasqua L,

Scorcia V, et al. Journal of Refractive Surgery. 2013;**29**(6):376-377

[28] Pahuja N, Shetty R, Jayadev C, Nuijts R, Hedge B, Arora V. Intraoperative optical coherence tomography using the RESCAN 700: Preliminary results in collagen crosslinking. BioMed Research International. 2014;**2015**:572698. DOI: 10.1155/2015/572698

Chapter 4

OCT Applications in Conjunctival Disease

Raffaele Piscopo, Michele Lanza, Luigi Mele and Mario Bifani Sconocchia

Abstract

Today the of anterior segment optical coherence tomography (ASOCT) has become an irreplaceable tool in the management of various pathologies and also in many surgical techniques. The cornea has been widely studied in many pathologies with ASOCT, but now also the conjunctival study with ASOCT allows to obtain a detailed imaging of the normal and pathological conjunctiva, so that in many conjunctival diseases the ASOCT is a useful tool to help the clinicians. In this chapter we will briefly discuss the results of the imaging of the oct appearance of the normal conjunctiva with ASOCT and its present and potential use in the conjunctival pathologies.

Keywords: anterior segment OCT, conjunctival diseases, conjunctiva, conjunctival tumors, optical coherence tomography

1. Introduction

The clinical application of ocular coherence tomography (OCT) and angio-OCT is today increasing and their use is not only focused on the retina so that, since the introduction of anterior OCT in the late 1990s, many other ocular pathologies of the eye have also been studied.

Today anterior segment OCT (ASOCT) is mainly used in corneal pathology since several years and its use is necessary in the management of the clinical and surgical activities [1–4].

Today there are different models of ASOCT and they can be mainly classified on the basis of the type of technology used to perform the scan: the time-domain technology, the spectral-domain technology, the swept source and, lately, also the angio-OCT study of the conjunctival and scleral vessel has been studied.

The aim and the ideal use of ASOCT in the anterior segment, especially in the conjunctiva, is to give an "optical biopsy" which can help the clinician in several ways: to distinguish among the various conjunctival tumors, to assess if a certain surgical technique has been effective or, in the future, to distinguish in the early stage between a neoplastic and inflammatory conjunctival disease.

The studies which discuss the use of such technologies have been focused on three main areas of interest: the characterization of the normal human conjunctiva with its possible variations, the use in the glaucoma filtering surgery and the study of the conjunctival pathologies.

2. Normal conjunctiva

The conjunctiva is composed of two layers: the epithelium and stroma. The epithelium consists of well-organized cell layers in both stratified squamous and columnar types. The stroma is a connective tissue of fibrous and vascular elements in a less organized disposition.

All these anatomy concepts have found a great correspondence in the OCT imaging, so that the aspect of the conjunctiva in the OCT image presents typical features as shown in several reports [5–10]. The use of ASOCT on the normal conjunctiva is a complete and useful tool since the OCT imaging already provides a detailed representation of healthy limbus, sclera and conjunctiva. These studies were mainly focused on evaluating the qualitative (the complete visualization of the anatomy) and quantitative (the thickness of the different stratus) aspects of this layer. The normal OCT appearance is shown in **Figure 1**, where it is possible to recognize a small hyporeflective zone (epithelium) on the top resting on a greater hyperreflective area (stroma and Tenon capsule). Differentiating among the various layers is easy thanks to the different brightness OCT features. The epithelium, consisting of well-aligned cell layers, results as hyporeflective part, because of the less scattering of the incident light from OCT.

The OCT image of the stroma is characterized by an higher brightness signal because of its different composition up above described: so this part of the tissue highly scatters the OCT incident light, thus it appears hyperreflective and clearly visible beneath the conjunctival epithelium.

The conjunctival stromal OCT characteristic is quite different from the corneal stroma, as reported in previous studies [9]: the superficial and deeper layers of the stroma are composed by an adenoid layer containing lymphocytes and mast cells laying on a fibrous layer which produces an increase in reflectivity.

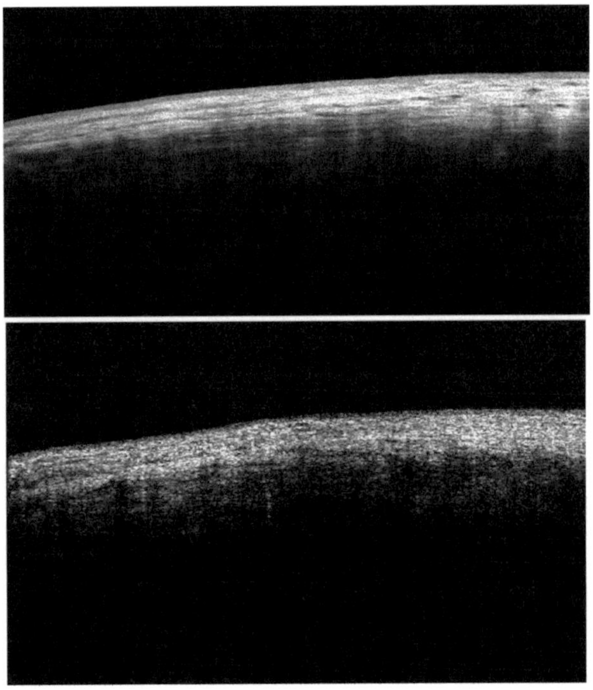

Figure 1.
Conjunctival OCT in a normal subject: the multistratified cylinder epithelium appears as a hyporeflective area, laid on a dense, hyperreflective connective layer. The lower reflective Tenon capsule is separated by a visible demarcation.

The underlying Tenon capsule has a high reflectivity similar to the conjunctival stroma in the OCT image. The distinction of these two layers is not always recognizable, possibly depending on the relationship between the stroma and the tenon: a clingy apposition near the limbus, for instance, makes the differentiation hard [7]. Thickness has been the most quantitative feature which has been studied: a detection of its variation could be an important sign of conjunctival health (edematous or thinning pathologies).

In their study, [7] Feng and Simpson reported the mean bulbar conjunctiva epithelial thickness was 44.9 ± 3.4 μm in 13 healthy subjects.

Another study reported the epithelial thickness being 42.0 ± 7.5 with a slight reduction in the group with a higher age [11], while also the stroma was measured to be about 240 (ranging from 140 to 304) in a report of 2013 [12].

A key concept is that significant variations in thickness may be found, mainly depending on the measurement locations (nasal, inferior, temporal or superior conjunctiva). These findings are consistent with the conjunctiva's anatomical characteristics: it is known that the stroma thickens in the fornix and thins at the limbus, but also differences in the different meridian have been shown in one report published by Read et al. [9].

The author demonstrated some interesting features:

- On average, the conjunctiva was significantly thicker in the nasal meridian (270 ± 90 μm) compared to the temporal meridian (mean thickness 249 ± 59 μm) ($p < 0.001$).

- The conjunctiva exhibited its minimum thickness at the scleral spur location (0 mm) for both the temporal (mean 218 ± 55 μm) and nasal meridians (mean 223 ± 40 μm); however, the pattern of change in thickness away from the scleral spur differed between the two meridians. For the temporal meridian, the conjunctiva increased to its maximum thickness at the 1 mm location (mean 267 ± 59 μm), whereas the nasal meridian exhibited its maximum thickness (mean 364 ± 122 μm) at the 4 mm location.

- The conjunctival thickness measures also showed some significant changes with age, reducing in thickness from childhood into early adulthood. These changes are reasonable if we consider histological studies demonstrating that the mucous layer (goblet cell density) reduces in early adulthood.

3. The use of oct in glaucoma

The evaluation of the postoperative effectiveness of glaucoma surgery is a well validated use of the anterior OCT [6, 8, 13].

The anterior OCT allows a detailed representation of the bleb architecture, giving information of the shape and functionality of a postsurgical bleb. Moreover, with ASOCT it is possible to observe if a bleb is functioning well and to know details about the wall and the internal architecture of the bleb.

Reports in literature show that there are a lot of aspects of the OCT conjunctival appearance which can be used to assess the functionality of the blebs: the internal aspect (diffuse or flat) [14], the internal bleb reflectivity (low reflectivity or high) or the wall thickness [15, 16].

There is also another interesting use described in literature, described by Mastropasqua et al.: the authors stated that the application of ASOCT for studying bleb modifications before and after bulbar massage is useful as it is possible to observe an increase of the bleb-wall thickness, intraepithelial microcysts, and the fluid-filled cavity area [13]. The study by Guthoff et al. [17], instead, analyzes the effect of the needling on the bleb ASOCT appearance.

4. The use of oct in Conjunctival pathologies

4.1 Conjunctival tumors

One of the most studied and validated applications of ASOCT regards conjunctival tumors.

Many reports [18–24] demonstrate that the OCT study of conjunctival tumors can help the clinician to: make the diagnosis, help to distinguish among different types of neoplasm or between benign and malign neoplasms, help to assess the follow up after the surgical excision of the tumor.

The classification of the conjunctival tumors may be summarised in the congenital and acquired lesions.

The acquired lesions can be distinguished in: pigmented and non-pigmented or, depending on the origin of the mass, in surface-epithelial, melanocytic, fibrous-vascular, myogenic, neural, lipomatous, lymphoid, histiocytic, leukemic or metastatic.

Essentially the most studied conjunctival lesions are the pigmented-melanocytic. This family of lesions includes nevus, racial melanosis, PAM (primary acquired melanosis) and melanoma. Among the non-melanocytic neoplastic lesions, the most frequently studied are squamous cell carcinoma and lymphoma.

4.1.1 Nevus

Nevus is the most common melanocytic tumor of the conjunctiva. It shows up as a discrete variably pigmented, slightly elevated sessile which usually remains quite stable during life with <1% risk of transformation into malignant melanoma. Histopathologically, a conjunctival nevus is composed of nests of benign melanocytes in the stroma near the basal layers of the epithelium.

A periodical follow-up, together with photographic comparison, is the best way to verify whether it is growing: sometimes you may need the mass excision if any growth is documented.

4.1.1.1 OCT appearance

The study of Shields et al. on 22 conjunctival nevi demonstrated that all margins of conjunctival nevi can be observed through ASOCT (high resolution in 100% of anterior borders and 82% of posterior borders). The sensitivity of AS-OCT for the detection of intrinsic cysts in a conjunctival nevus is 80%, its specificity is 100%, its positive predictive value is 100%, and its negative predictive value is 60% [22].

Regarding conjunctival nevi we can conclude that ASOCT seems to be more accurate in assessing the extent of these tumors as long as the nevus is not very thick and not heavily pigmented.

AS-OCT can also be used for differentiating a nevus from melanoma: unlike melanomas, the nevi usually contain intralesional cystic space (their presence usually confirms a chronic pathology) [21].

(Note that it is still debated whether the presence of cysts does not definitively rule out malignancy.)

4.1.2 Primary acquired melanosis (PAM)

Primary acquired melanosis, a frequent benign conjunctival pigmented lesion, can evolve into conjunctival melanoma. It is usually observed in middle-aged or elderly patients and, in contrast with conjunctival nevus, it is patchy, flat, and non-cystic and it is usually not well circumscribed. This lesion may arise with or without atypia, and the presence of the atypia leads to a 50% chance of melanoma [25].

4.1.2.1 OCT appearance

Histopathologically, PAM is characterized by the presence of abnormal melanocytes near the basal layer of the epithelium so the PAM ASOCT images is characterized by normal thickness but moderately hyperreflective basal epithelium with no invasion of the subepithelial space [21].

4.1.3 Squamous cell neoplasia

Squamous cell neoplasia may be classified in CIN or squamous cell carcinoma, depending on whether it presents as a localized lesion confined to the surface epithelium (conjunctival intraepithelial neoplasia or dysplasia) or as a more invasive pathology which has broken through the basement membrane and invaded the underlying stroma. (squamous cell carcinoma).

4.1.3.1 Conjunctival intraepithelial neoplasia (CIN)

CIN (others prefer the terms mild, moderate, or severe dysplasia) appears as a fleshy, sessile or minimally elevated lesion usually arising at the limbus in the interpalpebral fissure and less commonly in the forniceal or palpebral conjunctiva A white plaque (leukoplakia) may be present.

Histopathologically, it is characterized by the presence of immature abnormal cells. The several types of displasia depend on the presence of these abnormal epithelial cells which may partially (mild dysplasia), nearly fully (moderate dysplasia) or fully replace (severe dysplasia) the normal cells. Carcinoma-in-situ represents full thickness replacement by abnormal epithelial cells.

4.1.3.2 OCT appearance

Due to its epithelial onset, distinctive criteria of ASOCT are a thickened, hyper-reflective epithelial layer with an abrupt transition from normal to abnormal epithelium [23].

Shousha et al. [26] demonstrated that the use of UHR-OCT (ultra-high resolution OCT) in the diagnosis and follow-up of conjunctival and corneal intraepithelial neoplasia (CCIN) is possible.

In the different types of CIN the authors found thickened hyperreflective epithelium and abrupt transition from normal to hyperreflective epithelium. Their results demonstrated that macroscopically resolved residual tumor nodules can be visualized by UHR-OCT [26]. A disadvantage of UHR-OCT is that it is not high enough to assess intracellular characteristics.

4.1.4 Squamous cell carcinoma

As above mentioned, the SCC develops when the abnormal cells have invaded the stroma. Histopathologically, invasive squamous cell carcinoma is characterized by malignant squamous cells that have violated the basement membrane and have grown in sheets or cords into the stromal tissue.

4.1.4.1 OCT appearance

In the OCT imaging a squamous cell carcinoma is recognizable since the epithelium appears hyperreflective and thickened [27]. Several reports demonstrated that the ASOCT may be useful in the differentiation between SCC and similar lesions like amelanotic melanoma and corneal fibrosis or from pterygia with a very good correlation with histopathology [23, 26, 27]. HR-OCT can also be used for the monitoring of the resolution of SCC during therapy. In this way, HR-OCT can detect subtle residual epithelial thickening which is not visible on clinical examination [20].

4.1.5 Malignant melanoma

A Conjunctival is characterized by a high clinical variability. It may be pigmented and tan or, more generally, elevated conjunctival lesion, located in possible several parts of conjunctiva.

Histopathologically, conjunctival melanoma is composed of variably pigmented malignant melanocytes within the conjunctival stroma. Patients are typically 60–70 years old and present with a nodular mass arising either de novo, from a nevus, or from PAM with atypia [25]. Often prominent feeder vessels and surrounding flat PAM are present. Melanoma-related death rates are 5–17% at 5 years and 9–35% at 10 years, depending on the precursor lesion. Non-limbal locations portend a poorer prognosis. De novo melanomas tend to have the worst prognosis. Local recurrence is common and it can be 45% at 5 years and 59% at 10 years [25].

4.1.5.1 OCT appearance

AS-OCT images show a hyperreflective subepithelial lesion. The epithelium is a normal to slightly thick layer of epithelium with variable hyperreflectivity of the basal epithelium, which suggests some involvement of the epithelium with atypical melanocytes [21].

4.1.6 Conjunctival lymphoma

Conjunctiva lymphoma may appear as a diffuse, slightly elevated pink mass, termed “salmon patch.” The usual localization is at the fornix, usually hidden by the eyelid in the superior and inferior quadrants and not in the horizontal exposed parts of the bulbar conjunctiva or the limbus. Sometimes they arise from caruncle or plica semilunaris, but almost never in the palpebral conjunctiva.

The Oct appeareance: a recent published study [21] showed the AS-OCT appearance of the lesion, characterized by a normal layer of epithelium overlying homogeneous, dark, hyporeflective subepithelial lesions with smooth borders (**Figures 2** and **3**). The lesions can often contain monomorphic, stippled, dot-like infiltrates that correspond to the infiltration of monoclonal lymphocytes.

The author states that for both melanomas and lymphomas, ASOCT images do not always help the clinician obtain a definitive diagnosis as they do for OSSN, but can help guide the differential diagnosis. Nevertheless, the histopathologic analysis of tissue is needed for final confirmation.

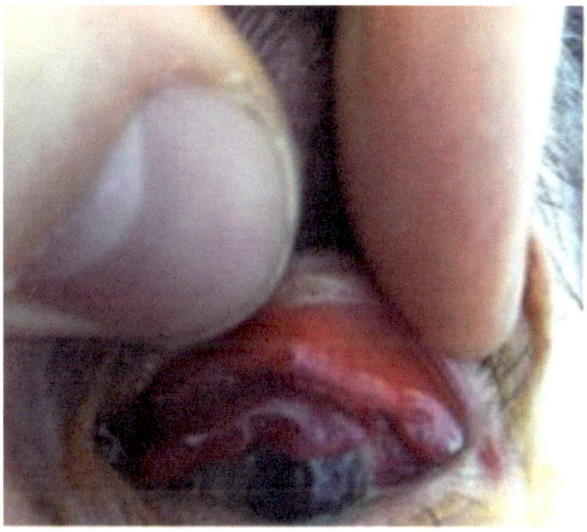

Figure 2.
Clinical appearance of conjunctival lymphoma.

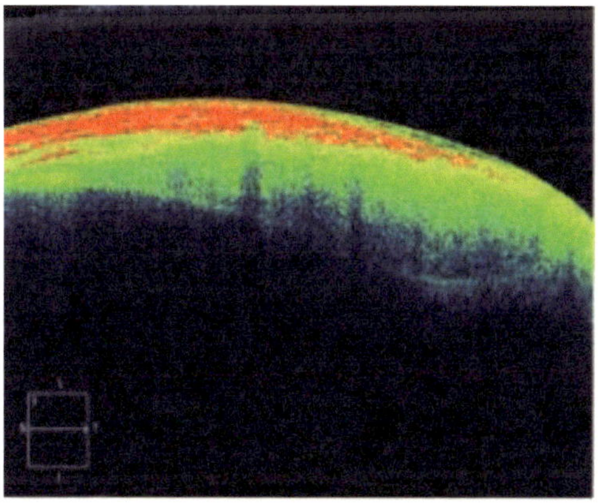

Figure 3.
OCT image: note the hyporeflective lesion with smooth posterior border.

4.2 Conjunctival diseases

4.2.1 Pterygium

In the pterygium the ASOCT can represent a useful tool if the corneal stromal invasion needs to be evaluated and also in the postoperative management.

ASOCT images of pterygia demonstrate a thin or normal layer of epithelium with varying levels of hyperreflectivity overlying a dense, hyperreflective, fibrillary subepithelial lesion that is between the corneal epithelium and Bowman's layer [21].

One of the aspects possibly involved in its recurrence is the pterygium length. Welch et al. studied the difference between the measurements of a pterygium using a slit-lamp or the ASOCT imaging. They demonstrated that ASOCT allows to accurately determine the extension of a pterygium on the cornea [28]. Moreover, ASOCT can help to distinguish pterygia from OSSN: various reports [18, 26–28] demonstrated statistically significant differences in epithelial thickness and location between these two lessons (thicker and epithelial for OSSN thinner and subepithelial for pterygia). Kieval et al. showed [27] that the average epithelial thickness in the 17 epithelial squamous cell carcinomas (SCC) was 346 μm, compared to 101 μm in the 17 pterygia. Using a cut-off value of 142 μm results in a sensitivity of 94% and a specificity of 100% in differentiating SCC from pterygia.

However, this imaging technique was less useful in evaluating pigmented lesions [20].

4.2.2 Graft-versus-host disease (GVHD)

Graft-versus-host disease (GVHD) is a major complication following allogeneic hematopoietic. It usually involves several organs, and the ocular involvement occurs in ~60% of GVHD patients [1, 3, 4], particularly affecting cornea, conjunctiva, lids and lacrimal gland, resulting in a wide spectrum of ocular complications [29–31] (**Figure 4**).

A report of Peng Li et al. [32] investigates the role of the device in GVHD with a surprising result: the conjunctival image of GVHD shows a characteristic imaging with a much higher OCT signal on the surface in GVHD patients compared to those in normal subjects (**Figure 5**), most likely due to the conjunctival keratinization and to the conjunctival lymphatic vessels dilated.

4.2.3 Ocular cicatricial pemphigoid

Mucous membrane pemphigoid (MMP) is an autoimmune, sub-epithelial blistering, potentially blinding disease characterized by scarring and shrinkage of mucosal membranes, including the conjunctival mucosa, oral cavity, esophagus, trachea and genitals [34]. When clinical signs are detected firstly in the conjunctiva, the disease is named "ocular cicatricial pemphigoid" (OCP) [33, 34] (**Figure 6**).

The diagnosis of ocular cicatricial pemphigoid (OCP) is challenging, especially when the pathology is in its early stages, due to the OCP a specific ocular signs which are not easy to recognize through slit lamp examination [35].

The ethiopathogenic mechanism by which the OCP produces its typical conjunctival lesions is a subepithelial inflammation mediated by autoimmunity against a multiplicities of possible antigens located in membrane basement of the deeper layers of the conjunctiva: this process leads t to a subconjunctival fibrosis and cicatricial conjunctivitis. Therefore, the ASOCT could potentially be a useful device to detect and study initial modifications of the conjunctival areas where OCP starts its damages, possibly when it is not recognizable by using the slit lamp alone. In our cohort of patients (unpublished data), we noticed in a great percentage some abnormalities in the OCT image: (**Figure 7**) a diffuse increase of optical reflectivity

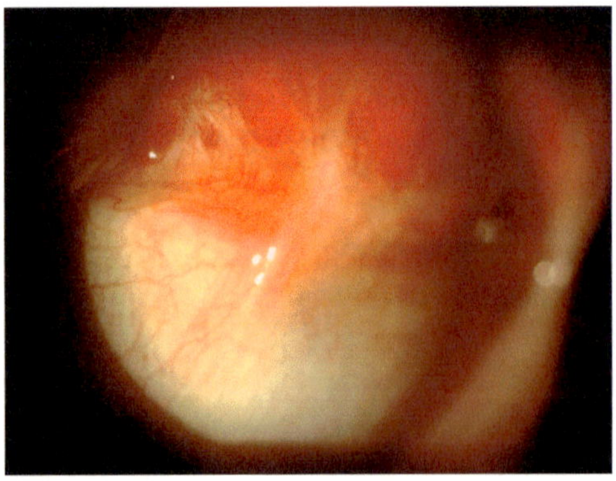

Figure 4.
Image of conjunctiva from a patient suffering from GVHD: a symblephara with the surrounding subepithelial fibrosis.

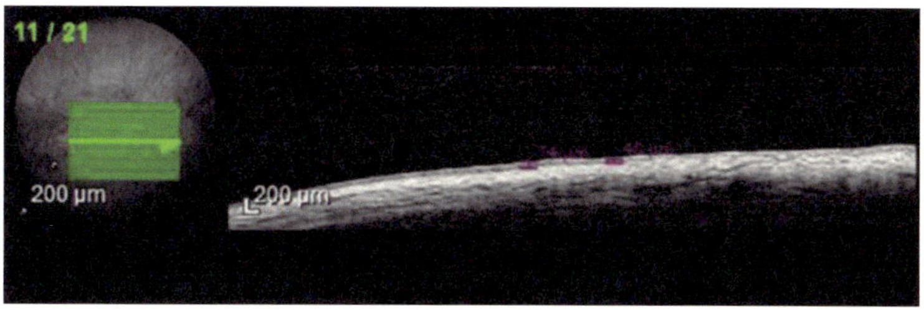

Figure 5.
OCT appearance of GVHD: diffuse hyperreflectivity of both epithelial and stromal area.

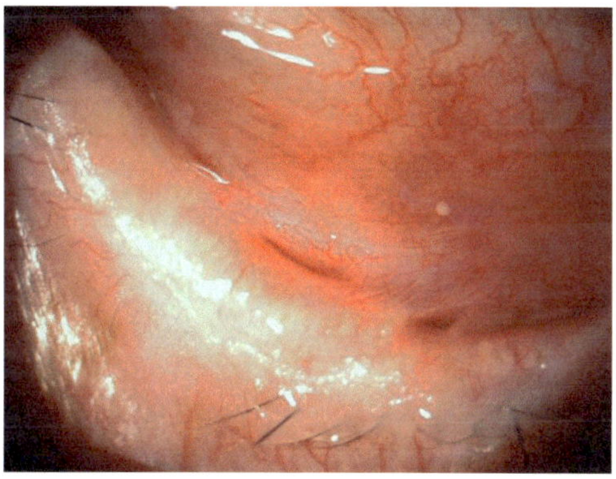

Figure 6.
Ocular cicatricial pemphigoid: note the fornix foreshortening and symblephara.

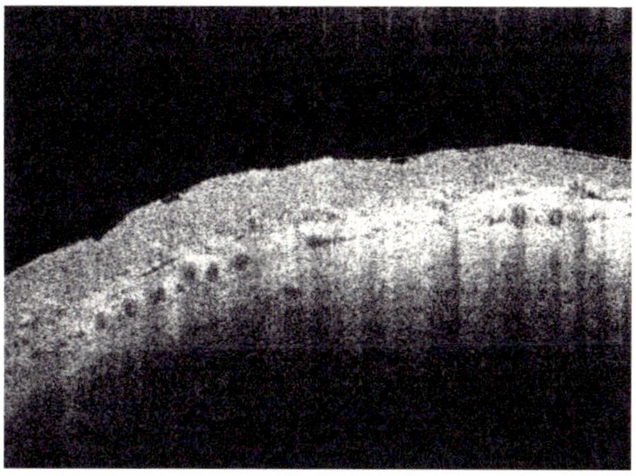

Figure 7.
*OCT appearance of the patient in **Figure 6**.*

located in the sub-epithelial conjunctival space and the presence of some folds located at different depths in the conjunctival substantia propria thickness, appearing in different shapes. These signs are usually located in the subepithelial space (distance 25 ± 8 µm from epithelium).

Conflict of interest

None of the authors have conflict of interest.

Author details

Raffaele Piscopo[1*], Michele Lanza[2], Luigi Mele[2] and Mario Bifani Sconocchia[2]

1 Eye Center, Humanitas Research Hospital, Milan, Italy

2 Multidisciplinary Department of Medical, Surgical and Dental Sciences, Second University of Napoli, Napoli, Italy

*Address all correspondence to: raffaele.piscopo@humanitas.it

References

[1] Werkmeister RM, Stegmann H, Dos Santos VA, Schmidl D, Schmetterer L. Cornea imaging by optical coherence tomography—Historical aspects and most recent technical developments. Klinische Monatsblätter für Augenheilkunde. 2018;**235**(12):1342-1351. DOI: 10.1055/a-0749-8947. Epub 19 December 2018. German

[2] Gumus K, Pflugfelder SC. Anterior segment optical coherence tomography (AS-OCT) in the management of dry eye. International Ophthalmology Clinics. 2017;**57**(2):13-22. DOI: 10.1097/IIO.0000000000000164. Review

[3] Abdelazeem K, Sharaf M, Saleh MGA, Fathalla AM, Soliman W. Relevance of swept-source anterior segment optical coherence tomography for corneal imaging in patients with flap-related complications after LASIK. Cornea. 2019;**38**(1):93-97. DOI: 10.1097/ICO.0000000000001773

[4] Petrovic A, Gianniou C, Hashemi K, Kymionis G. Intraoperative anterior optical coherence tomography-guided synechiolysis in a post-penetrating keratoplasty patient with peripheral corneal opacification. Therapeutics and Clinical Risk Management. 2018;**14**:1387-1390. DOI: 10.2147/TCRM.S167025. eCollection 2018

[5] Sridhar MS, Martin R. Anterior segment optical coherence tomography for evaluation of cornea and ocular surface. Indian Journal of Ophthalmology. 2018;**66**(3):367-372. DOI: 10.4103/ijo.IJO_823_17. Review

[6] Kuerten D, Plange N, Becker J, Walter P, Fuest M. Evaluation of long-term anatomic changes following canaloplasty with anterior segment spectral-domain optical coherence tomography and ultrasound biomicroscopy. Journal of Glaucoma. 2018;**27**(1):87-93. DOI: 10.1097/IJG.0000000000000827

[7] Feng Y, Simpson TL. Corneal, limbal, and conjunctival epithelial thickness from optical coherence tomography. Optometry and Vision Science. 2008;**85**(9):E880-E883

[8] Heisler M, Quong WL, Lee S, Han S, Beg MF, Sarunic MV, et al. Anterior segment optical coherence tomography for targeted transconjunctival suture placement in over filtering trabeculectomy blebs. Journal of Glaucoma. 2017;**26**(5):486-490. DOI: 10.1097/IJG.0000000000000656

[9] Read SA, Alonso-Caneiro D, Vincent SJ, Bremner A, Fothergill A, Ismail B, et al. Anterior eye tissue morphology: Scleral and conjunctival thickness in children and young adults. Scientific Reports. 2016;**6**:33796. DOI: 10.1038/srep33796

[10] Zhang X, Li Q, Liu B, Zhou H, Wang H, Zhang Z, et al. In vivo cross-sectional observation and thickness measurement of bulbar conjunctiva using optical coherence tomography. Investigative Ophthalmology and Visual Science. 2011;**52**:7787-7791

[11] Francoz M, Karamoko I, Baudouin C, Labbe A. Ocular surface epithelial thickness evaluation with spectral-domain optical coherence tomography. Investigative Ophthalmology and Visual Science. 2011;**52**:9116-9123

[12] Zhang X, Li Q, et al. Bulbar conjunctival thickness measurements with optical coherence tomography in healthy Chinese subjects. Investigative Ophthalmology & Visual Science. 2013;**54**:4705-4709. DOI: 10.1167/iovs.12-11003

[13] Mastropasqua R, Fasanella V, Agnifili L, Curcio C, Ciancaglini M, Mastropasqua L. Anterior segment optical coherence tomography imaging of conjunctival filtering blebs after

glaucoma surgery. BioMed Research International. 2014;**2014**:610623. DOI: 10.1155/2014/610623. Epub 20 July 2014

[14] Leung CK, Yick DW, Kwong YY, et al. Analysis of bleb morphology after trabeculectomy with Visante anterior segment optical coherence tomography. British Journal of Ophthalmology. 2007;**91**(3):340-344

[15] Pfenninger L, Schneider F, Funk J. Internal reflectivity of filtering blebs versus intraocular pressure in patients with recent trabeculectomy. Investigative Ophthalmology and Visual Science. 2011;**52**(5):2450-2455

[16] Tominaga A, Miki A, Yamazaki Y, Matsushita K, Otori Y. The assessment of the filtering bleb function with anterior segment optical coherence tomography. Journal of Glaucoma. 2010;**19**(8):551-555

[17] Guthoff R, Guthoff T, Hensler D, Grehn F, Klink T. Bleb needling in encapsulated filtering blebs: Evaluation by optical coherence tomography. Ophthalmologica. 2010;**224**(4):204-208

[18] Thomas BJ, Galor A, Nanji AA, El Sayyad F, Wang J, Dubovy SR, et al. Ultra high-resolution anterior segment optical coherence tomography in the diagnosis and management of ocular surface squamous neoplasia. The Ocular Surface. 2014;**12**(1):46-58. DOI: 10.1016/ Epub 2013 Nov9

[19] Vizvári E, Skribek Á, Polgár N, Vörös A, Sziklai P, Tóth-Molnár E. Conjunctival melanocytic naevus: Diagnostic value of anterior segment optical coherence tomography and ultrasound biomicroscopy. PLoS ONE. 2018;**13**(2):e0192908. DOI: 10.1371/journal.pone.0192908

[20] Janssens K, Mertens M, Lauwers N, de Keizer RJ, Mathysen DG, De Groot V. To study and determine the role of anterior segment optical coherence tomography and ultrasound biomicroscopy in corneal and conjunctival tumors. Journal of Ophthalmology. 2016;**2016**:1048760. DOI: 10.1155/2016/1048760. Epub 6 December 2016

[21] Venkateswaran N, Galor A, Wang J, Karp CL. Optical coherence tomography for ocular surface and corneal diseases: A review. Eye and Vision. 2018;**5**:13

[22] Shields CL, Belinsky I, Romanelli-Gobbi M, et al. Anterior segment optical coherence tomography of conjunctival nevus. Ophthalmology. 2011;**118**(5):915-919

[23] Nanji AA, Sayyad FE, Galor A, Dubovy S, Karp CL. High-resolution optical coherence tomography as an adjunctive tool in the diagnosis of corneal and conjunctival pathology. The Ocular Surface. 2015;**13**(3):226-235

[24] Bianciotto C, Shields CL, Guzman JM, et al. Assessment of anterior segment tumors with ultrasound biomicroscopy versus anterior segment optical coherence tomography in 200 cases. Ophthalmology. 2011;**118**(7):1297-1302

[25] Shields CL, Shields JA. Tumors of the conjunctiva and cornea. Survey of Ophthalmology. 2004;**49**(1):3-24. DOI: 10.1016/j.survophthal.2003.10.008

[26] Shousha MA, Karp CL, Perez VL, et al. Diagnosis and management of conjunctival and corneal intraepithelial neoplasia using ultra high-resolution optical coherence tomography. Ophthalmology. 2011;**118**(8):1531-1537

[27] Kieval JZ, Karp CL, Shoushaetal MA. Ultra-high resolution optical coherence tomography for differentiation of ocular surface squamous neoplasia and pterygia. Ophthalmology. 2012;**119**(3):481-486

[28] Welch MN, Reilly CD, Kalwerisky K, Johnson A, Waller SG. Pterygia measurements are more accurate with anterior segment optical coherence tomography—A pilot study. Nepalese Journal of Ophthalmology. 2011;**3**(1):9-12

[29] Qiu Y, Hong J, Peng R. Manifestation of clinical categories of ocular graft-versus-host disease. Journal of Ophthalmology. 2018;**2018**:6430953. DOI: 10.1155/2018/6430953 eCollection 2018

[30] Lauermann JL, Treder M, Stelljes M, Groth C, Eter N, Uhlig CE. Bilateral corneal calcification in ocular graft-versus-host disease. Der Ophthalmologe. Feb 2019;**116**(2):185-188. DOI: 10.1007/s00347-018-0695-z. [Epub ahead of print] German

[31] Berchicci L, Rabiolo A, Marchese A, Iuliano L, Gigliotti C, Miserocchi E, et al. Ocular chronic graft-versus-host disease after allogeneic hematopoietic stem cell transplantation in an Italian referral center. The Ocular Surface. 2018;**16**(3):314-321. DOI: 10.1016/j.jtos.2018.04.001. Epub 4 April 2018

[32] Li P, Sun Y, Hariri S, Zhou Z, Inamoto Y, Lee SJ, et al. Wang. Anterior segment optical coherence tomography evaluation of ocular graft-versus-host disease: A case study. Quantitative Imaging in Medicine and Surgery. 2015;**5**(1):163-170. DOI: 10.3978/j.issn.2223-4292.2014.11.05

[33] Günther C. Involvement of mucous membranes in autoimmune bullous diseases. Der Hautarzt. 2016;**67**(10):774-779. Review. German

[34] Wang K, Seitzman G, Gonzales JA. Ocular cicatricial pemphigoid. Current Opinion in Ophthalmology. 2018;**29**(6):543-551. DOI: 10.1097/ICU.0000000000000517

[35] Dart JK. The 2016 Bowman lecture conjunctival curses: Scarring conjunctivitis 30 years on. Eye (London, England). 2017;**31**(2):301-332. DOI: 10.1038/eye.2016.284. Epub 20 January 2017

Section 2

OCT in Retinal Diseases

Chapter 5

New Landmarks, Signs, and Findings in Optical Coherence Tomography

Francisco Javier Lara-Medina, Olivia Esteban, Isabel Bartolomé, C. Ispa, Javier Mateo and Francisco Javier Ascaso

Abstract

Spectral domain optical coherence tomography (SD-OCT) is a common useful noninvasive imaging instrument which is used for the diagnosis and follow-up of macular disorders. The clinical findings by OCT in these pathologies are well known. Currently, due to the development of this technology and its wide use, new OCT findings have been reported in the literature. The aim of this chapter is to describe new pathological or abnormal signs and findings in SD-OCT, including hyperreflective spots or dots, flyer saucer sign, outer retinal tubulations, dipping sign, focal choroidal excavation, outer retina-choroid complex splitting, foveal pseudocyst, brush border pattern, dome-shaped macula, pearl necklace sign, choroidal macrovessel, cystoid foveal degeneration, and disorganization of the retinal inner layers (DRIL).

Keywords: hyperreflective spots, perifoveal cupping, flyer saucer sign, tubulations, dipping sign, outer retina-choroid complex splitting, foveal pseudocyst, brush border pattern, dome-shaped macula, pearl necklace sign, macrovessel, disorganization of the retinal inner layers

1. Introduction

Spectral domain optical coherence tomography (SD-OCT) is a common useful noninvasive imaging instrument which is used for the diagnosis and follow-up of macular diseases, such as age-related macular degeneration (AMD), diabetic macular edema (DME), epiretinal membrane (ERM), or macular hole. The clinical findings by OCT in these pathologies are well known. SD-OCT allows detail assessment of the retinal thickness and morphologic evaluation of the retinal layers. Currently, due to the development of this technology and its extensive use, new OCT findings have been reported in the literature. The higher resolution and speed of SD-OCT have improved the accuracy and reproducibility of macular imaging and have allowed an enhanced assessment of the integrity of the outer retinal bands.

IntechOpen

2. New landmarks in OCT

OCT imaging is similar to ultrasonography, except that it uses infrared light reflections instead of acoustic waves. The OCT image is displayed using a false color map that corresponds to detected backscattered light levels from the incident light. White and red colors represent high reflectivity signals, while the low reflectivity signals correspond to black and blue colors [1]. OCT interpretations make necessary knowledge of the normal anatomy of the retina. In a usual SD-OCT scan, a highly scattering layer delineates the posterior boundary of the retina and corresponds to the retinal pigment epithelium (RPE) and choriocapillaris complex. The nerve fiber layer is manifest as a highly backscattering red layer at the vitreoretinal interface. Both layers are the posterior and anterior boundaries of the sensory retina and are essential to quantify the neurosensorial retinal thickness [2]. The rest of the layers of the neurosensorial retina are disposed between the two limits, and they are observed with OCT in a similar way to a histological section. The high reflectivity signal (yellow and red colors) come from the retinal nerve fiber layer (RNFL), inner plexiform layer, outer plexiform layer (OPL), internal limiting membrane (ILM), junction between inner and outer segments of photoreceptors (IS/OS), and RPE and choriocapillaris complex. The low reflectivity signals (black and blue colors) correspond to the nuclear layers [3]. In 2014, an international panel of OCT experts agreed on the adequate nomenclature for the retinal layers as visualized on OCT [4]. The new terminology of the outer retinal bands and their anatomical correspondence are described below, from the innermost to the outermost (**Figure 1**) [4, 5]:

1. The external limiting membrane band (ELM) is located at the boundary between the nuclei (cell bodies) and the inner segments of the photoreceptors and comprises clusters of junctional complexes between the Müller cells and the photoreceptors.

2. The ellipsoid zone (EZ), which was previously referred as the photoreceptor inner segment/outer segment (IS/OS) junction, is considered to be formed mainly by mitochondria within the ellipsoid layer of the outer portion of the inner segments of the photoreceptors. In a normal fovea, the distance from the EZ line to the ELM line is shorter than that from the EZ line to the RPE. The EZ "elevation" in the foveal center is due to elongated foveal cone outer segments.

3. The interdigitation zone (IZ) is considered to be the contact cylinders formed by the apices of the RPE cells that encase the part of the cone outer segments. This layer is not always recognizable from the underlying RPE layer, even in healthy subjects.

4. The retinal pigment epithelial band is formed by the RPE and Bruch's membrane. Both structures are indistinguishable from each other using the currently commercial SD-OCT. In the fovea, this band is thicker compared to other regions, which indicates that choroidal structures may also participate in the hyperreflectivity of the RPE band at this location.

Recent publications have reported that the damage or the alteration of the photoreceptors supposes a loss of integrity of some of these four bands previously described [6, 7]. Series of OCT images in different phases of degenerative diseases of the retina have demonstrated that IZ, EZ, and ELM lengths are highly correlated with each other. The affectation seems to occur in a stepwise sequence: first at the

DOI: http://dx.doi.org/10.5772/intechopen.84242

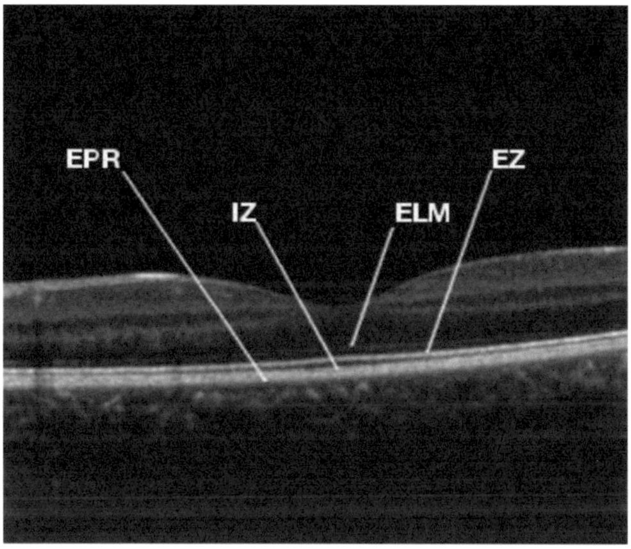

Figure 1.
Spectral domain optical coherence tomography (SD-OCT) scan with external retinal landmarks from a healthy subject. RPE: retina pigment epithelium; IZ: interdigitation zone; EZ: ellipsoid zone; and ELM: external limiting membrane.

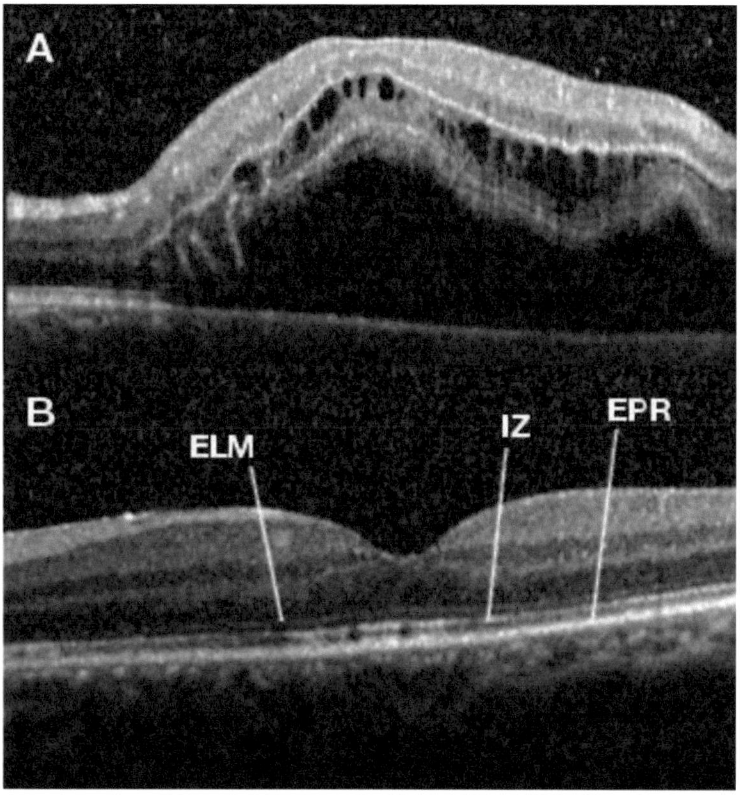

Figure 2.
SD-OCT in a patient with retinal detachment macula off (A). Post-surgical aspect through OCT of the same patient in which the integrity of the outer layers is observed (B). The visual acuity was 20/30.

IZ, followed by the EZ, and finally the ELM band [7–9]. Similarly, photoreceptor restoration seems to occur in the reverse order. After closing a macular hole, it has been documented that the ELM zone is the first structure to recover, and its recovery has been considered a sign of intact Müller cells and photoreceptor cell bodies [10]. Also, OCT findings after ERM and macular hole surgeries showed that recovery of EZ line only occurred in areas with intact ELM, and IZ recovery was only observed in eyes with EZ and ELM uninjured [11, 12]. The recovery of the ELM line following treatment has been correlated with visual acuity outcomes for macular hole [11, 13], retinal detachment [9], and AMD [14]. After macular hole closure, the presence of injured ELM was associated with reduced visual acuity [12]. In retinal detachment (RD), preservation of the ELM line postoperatively was related with better visual acuity result and also seems to predict the subsequent restoration of the photoreceptor layer [9]. Disruption or absence of the EZ line has been shown to correlate with visual acuity and severity in several retinal diseases [5]. In non-neovascular AMD, disruption of the EZ has been associated with visual impairment [15–17]. Furthermore, retinal sensitivity in patients with geographic atrophy was significantly higher in areas with an uninjured EZ [18]. In neovascular AMD, intact EZ at baseline was reported as a favorable prognostic factor for visual acuity outcome following intravitreal anti-vascular endothelium growth factor (anti-VEGF) treatment [14]. In diabetic patients with macular edema, the EZ disruption at the fovea was reported as a significant predictor of visual acuity [19, 20]. In eyes with ERM, preoperative disruptions of the EZ line were also associated with poorer visual acuity outcomes [21–23]. The IZ line is very difficult to identify even in healthy subjects. A correlation between the postoperative status of IZ and visual acuity has been described for macular hole [11], ERM [21], and RD [24]. Gharbiya and collaborators reported that the integrity of the IZ line was the strongest predictor of visual acuity outcome after primary RD repair (**Figure 2**) [24]. Following macular hole surgery, patients with irregular or discrete IZ line had significantly better visual acuity compared with those eyes with a disrupted or absent IZ line at the one-year visit follow-up [14]. In recent years, new OCT findings and signs have been reported for different retinal diseases. We will describe them with more clinical relevance.

3. New findings and signs

3.1 Hyperreflective retinal spots (HRS)

Coscas and cols were the first authors to report the presence of HRS on SD-OCT in exudative AMD [25]. These dots are described as small in size (20–40 μm in diameter), punctiform hyperreflective elements (equal or higher reflectivity than the RPE band), distributed throughout all retinal layers. HRS are mainly located at the border of the ONL and within the OPL [26]. They have also been reported in early stages of DR and also in diabetics without any clinical sign of DR, DME, retinal venous occlusion (RVO), central serous chorioretinopathy (CSCR), macular telangiectasias, and certain types of uveitis (**Figure 3**) [27]. It has been hypothesized that HRS represent aggregates of microglial activated cells and could indicate a retinal inflammatory response. Therefore, it has been reported reduction of HRS number following intravitreal anti-VEGF or dexamethasone therapies [28]. There are various theories on the pathogenesis of HRS. Some authors hypothesize that HRS are focal pigment accumulations of lipofuscin granules. Others consider that there could be small intraretinal protein or lipid deposits/exudates secondary to the breakdown of the blood-retinal barrier in retinal vascular diseases [26–30]. According to other theory, HRS might be derived from the degenerated photoreceptors or from the macrophages that

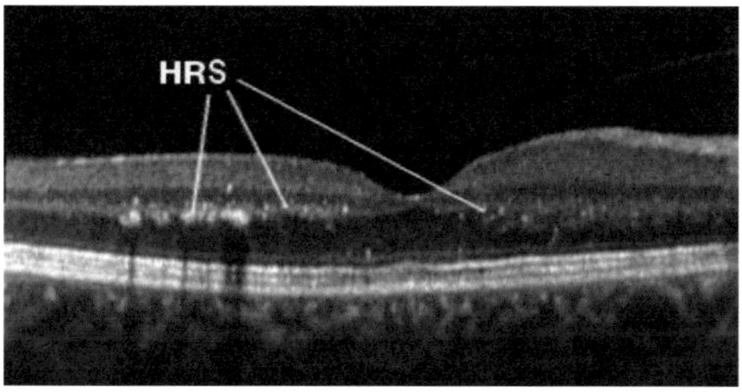

Figure 3.
Hyperreflective retinal spots (HRS) observed in a patient affected of tuberculosis posterior uveitis.

phagocyted them [31]. Concerning the clinical implications of the HRS, we have already commented that they represent a certain degree of retinal inflammation. HRS are associated with poorer visual outcome in patients with macular edema due to retinal vascular diseases such as RD or RVO. The therapeutic response to specific treatments might be different according to the number of HRS. Hwang et al. reported an inadequate response to intravitreal bevacizumab for DME and macular edema due to RVO in eyes with a greater number of HRS. Eyes that responded poorly to bevacizumab were treated with dexamethasone implants. About 75% of such eyes showed a good response and corresponded to the eyes with a higher number of HRS [32]. Vujosevic and cols have also suggested that DME with a high number of HRS and a large area of increased foveal autofluorescence showed better morphologic and functional results (better retinal sensitivity) if, at least initially, was treated with intravitreal steroids versus anti-VEGF [28]. These findings suggest that in eyes with several HRS, the inflammatory pathway might contribute to the pathogenesis of the macular edema more than the VEGF pathway. Therefore, in patients with macular edema and many HRS, anti-inflammatory drugs (e.g., dexamethasone intravitreal implant) might be more effective than intravitreal anti-VEGF treatment [32].

3.2 Flying saucer sign

The use of hydroxychloroquine (HCQ), an antimalarial drug utilized for a range of rheumatologic and dermatologic diseases, is associated with a low incidence of retinopathy (1% after 5 years) when used at recommended doses (<6.5 mg/kg/day) [33]. However, the retinopathy described as a bull's-eye is untreatable and tends to progress even after cessation of the drug. In recent years, there is an increased interest in screening by using multimodal imaging techniques to detect early signs of retinal toxicity. SD-OCT may detect significant structural alterations before the development of visible HCQ retinopathy. Several OCT findings have been described in the literature such as disruption of the EZ line, loss of the ELM, parafoveal thinning of the ONL, and RPE damage. These studies suggest that there is a foveal resistance to HCQ damage as demonstrated by the preservation of the subfoveal outer retinal layers. This foveal sparing originates the "flying saucer" sign on HCQ retinopathy (**Figure 4**) [34]. The main characteristics of this sign include the loss of the normal foveal depression, perifoveal thinning of the ONL, an ovoid appearance of the central fovea, conservation of the outer retinal structures and photoreceptor IS/OS junction in the central fovea, an apparent posterior displacement of the inner retinal structures toward RPE, and perifoveal loss of the photoreceptor IS/OS junction [3]. All these alterations originate an ovoid appearance in the central fovea [35]. This sign is neither pathognomonic nor necessary for the diagnosis of HCQ

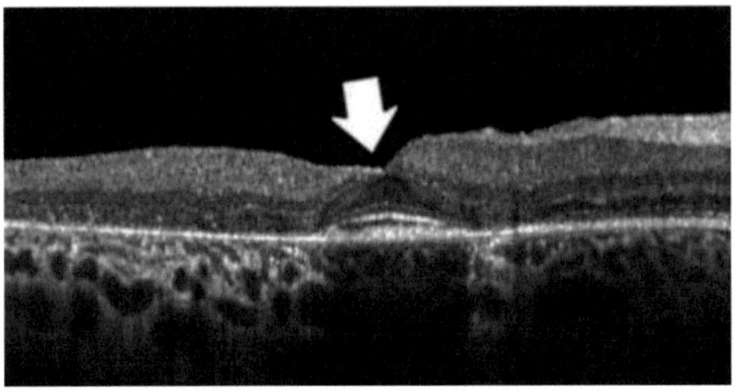

Figure 4.
SD-OCT revealed the "flying saucer" sign in a woman treated with oral chloroquine at a dosage of 3 mg/kg once daily for 8 years.

retinopathy. Nevertheless, its visualization on SD-OCT images should alert us to possible retinal toxicity due to HCQ toxicity.

3.3 Outer retinal tubulation (ORT)

ORT is a degenerative process of outer retinal reorganization located primarily in eyes where the macula is disrupted and RPE is absent. ORTs are ovoid or circular hyporeflective lesions surrounded by a hyperreflective ring always located in the ONL in eyes with advanced outer retinal diseases (**Figure 5**) [36]. It has been described in numerous retinal disorders showing macular atrophy involving RPE, such as AMD [36], mitochondrial diseases [37], and retinal dystrophies [38]. They have also been reported in cases of macular neovascularization including AMD, choroidal nevus, pseudoxanthoma elasticum [39], multifocal choroiditis with uveitis and CNMV, choroideremia [36], and enhanced S-cone syndrome [40]. Histologic studies showed interconnecting tubes of surviving cone photoreceptors interleaved with and contained by processes of Müller cells [41]. Histologically, the hyperreflective border of ORS seen in SD-OCT images corresponds with the presence of both an EML delimiting the lumen and mitochondria migrating from the inner segments to the cell bodies of degenerating cone photoreceptor. The main histologic characteristics of ORTs are [41]:

1. location at the level of ONL

2. presence of an ELM surrounding all or part of the lumen

3. presence of enclosing radially oriented photoreceptors pointing to the lumen

4. disruption or absence of the underlying RPE

There are different shapes of ORTs: open, closed, forming, and branching. A branching or pseudodendritic pattern is observed mainly in macular neovascularization, whereas a single tube is more frequent in the border of geographic atrophy [42]. Regarding the etiology of these tubulations, it has been hypothesized to be related to the different shapes of the ELM descent (flat, curved, and reflected). As the RPE begins to atrophy, the ELM descent changes from flat to curved, then reflected to scrolled, and finally, an area of ORT may appear. In this process, Müller cells expand and fill the spaces created by the loss of photoreceptors, as they are the only structure persisting in end-stage of ORT. The presence of a scrolled ELM descent may represent a predictive factor for progression toward ORT. It has been reported that in cases of neovascularization, the progression to ORT experienced a shorter period between

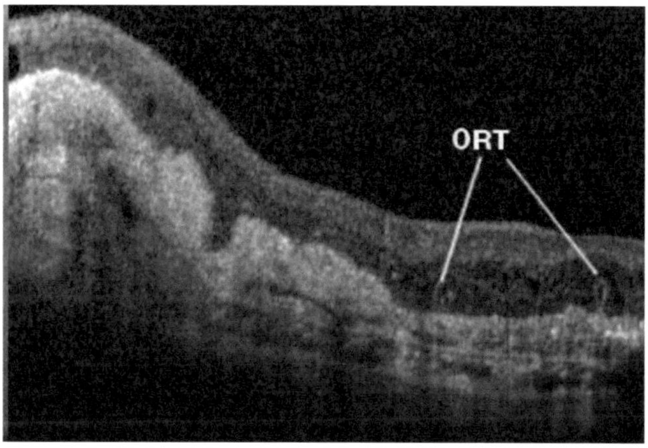

Figure 5.
Outer external tabulation in atrophic age-macular degeneration.

the steps of flat and curved ELM than eyes only with atrophic [42]. ORTs have a significant prognostic value since their presence suggests a poor visual acuity. They should be differentiated from intraretinal or subretinal fluid cysts located at the outer retinal layers. Intraretinal fluid cysts in cystoid macular edema (CME) have the arrangement as a petaloid manner, while ORTs are randomly arranged at the macula. Pseudocysts are usually distinguished from ORTs because they are located in the inner nuclear layer. Retinal tubulations are always located at the level of the ONL [3]. ORTs are circular hyporeflective lesions surrounded by a hyperreflective ring. This hyperreflective border is absent in cysts. Likewise, ORTs may contain a few focal hyperreflective spots in contrast to the completely hyporeflective cystoid lesions. The recognition of ORT may avoid unnecessary treatment because it is more refractory to anti-VEGF treatment compared to the cysts. Because outer tubulations tend to change slowly over time, it is unlikely to be associated with an active exudative or inflammatory process. For that reason, they do not require treatment [3, 42]. ORT can also be differentiated from rosettes described in retinoblastoma by their large size, tubular structure, and degenerative instead of developmental nature. In retinitis pigmentosa, there are also rosettes which are distinguished from ORTs by their location outside the macula and absence of degeneration of the underlying RPE [42].

3.4 Dome-shaped macula

Dome-shaped macula (DSM) is an inward protrusion of the macula as visualized by OCT (**Figure 6**). Different patterns have been described by OCT: a horizontal or vertical oval-shaped dome and a round dome [43]. DSM was first reported in myopic eyes with posterior staphyloma, but more recently has also been described

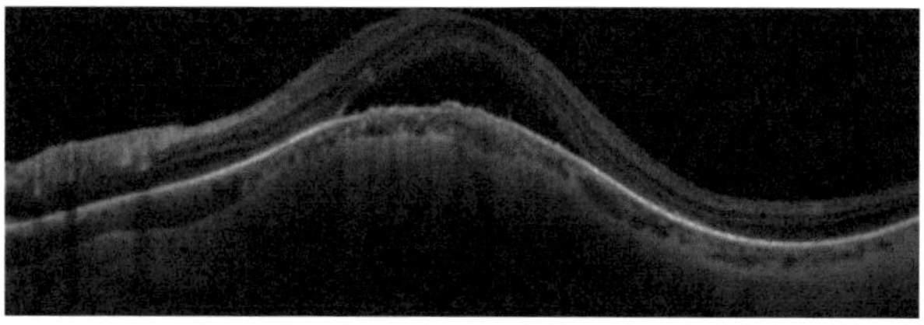

Figure 6.
SD-OCT showing a dome-shaped macula.

in patients without staphyloma, emmetropic, or hypermetropic eyes [44, 45]. A variety of hypotheses have been postulated to explain it: an adaptive mechanism to minimize defocus in highly myopic eyes [46], vitreomacular traction [47], ocular hypotony [47], resistance of the sclera to the staphylomatous deformation [48], or localized choroidal thickening [48]. However, it has been recently indicated that the main problem is the different degrees of scleral thinning in the foveal region [46, 49, 50]. Subretinal fluid (SRF) in the fovea has been associated continuously with DSM in 28.5–66.6% of patients [51]. It may be due to RPE dysfunction [48] or as a consequence of not uniform scleral thickness that can affect choroidal fluid [46]. Although photodynamic therapy and anti-VEGF agents have been applied, they had no effects in terms of improvement in BCVA and resolution of SRF, because the fluid remained chronic and stable in most of the eyes over time [51], and it was even spontaneously resolved in 47% of the cases [52].

3.5 Brush border pattern or elongation of photoreceptor outer segment

Brush border pattern is defined as an accumulation of waste products in the photoreceptor outer segment on the outer surface of the detached neurosensory retina over subretinal fluid (**Figure 7**). This provides an irregular, serrated, and thicker appearance of the detached neurosensory retina. Other authors denominate it as "elongation of the outer photoreceptor segment", and it can be found in almost 73–75% of OCT images from patients who suffer CSCR [53]. The loss of the contact between RPE and photoreceptor outer segments that occur in CSCR prevents the waste product of photoreceptors being phagocytosed by RPE [54]. These subretinal proteins or accumulated macrophages with outer photoreceptor segments can be observed as hyperfluorescent white-yellowish precipitates in the retinal examination if they contain precursors of lipofuscin [55]. If this process persists, despite subretinal fluid absorption, subretinal deposits may progress to be permanent with the subsequent poor visual outcome. Complete disappearance of outer segments as observed in very long-standing CSCR correlates with poor visual prognosis [53].

3.6 Outer retina-choroid complex (ORCC) splitting

Patients at intermediate clinical stages in Best vitelliform macular dystrophy (BVMD) show split in the ORCC by OCT. The ORCC has multiple components, and it is split into subcomponents showing different patterns [56]. Such patterns of ORCC splitting represent the separation between the apical surface of the RPE and photoreceptors causing neurosensory macular retinal detachment (**Figure 8**) [57]. OCT shows a diffuse, irregular, and thickened ORCC by underlying hyporeflective area [3].

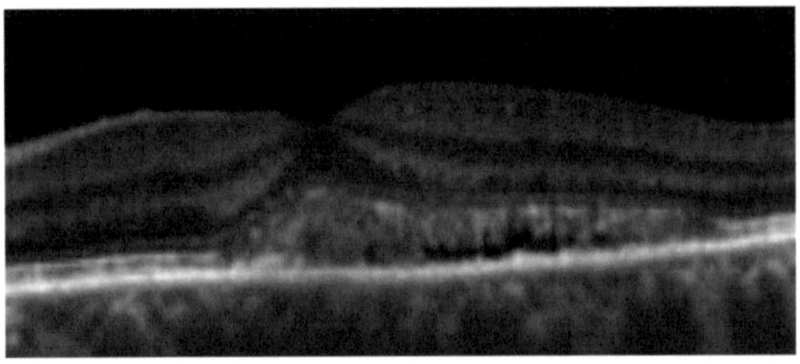

Figure 7.
Brush border pattern in patient affected of chronic central serous chorioretinopathy (CSCR).

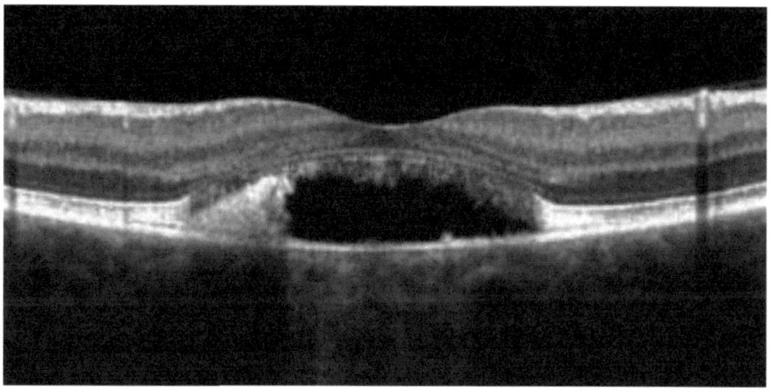

Figure 8.
SD-OCT shows a splitting of outer retina-choroid complex by hyporeflective area in a patient with Best vitelliform macular dystrophy.

3.7 Disorganization of retinal inner layers (DRIL)

DRIL is observed on OCT as the difficulty to identify limits between the ganglion cell-inner plexiform layer complex, inner nuclear layer, and OPL (**Figure 9**). It represents an interrupted transmission pathway between the photoreceptors and ganglion cells due to the disruptions of synaptic connections of amacrine, bipolar, and horizontal cells [58]. Several hypotheses explain the pathogenesis: **mechanical factor** (stretching of bipolar axons by edema) and **vascular factors** (ischemia, loss of the retinal capillary plexuses, or neuroglial degeneration as sequelae of inflammation) [58–62]. DRIL has been described as a strong predictive factor of worse visual acuity in patients with DME [58], uveitic macular edema [63], and central retinal vein occlusion [64]. Although the role of ischemia in DRIL is being studied, authors have found that areas of macular capillary nonperfusion were strongly correlated with DRIL on fluorescein angiography (FA) in severe nonproliferative and proliferative diabetic retinopathy (PDR) [59]. Moreover, more recently, OCT angiography has allowed researchers to study the positive correlation between DRIL and the size of the foveal avascular zone in diabetic retinopathy and retinal vein occlusion [60, 65]. Even, it has been associated with higher body mass index, longer diabetes duration, and increasing severity of PDR [66, 67]. Several studies have demonstrated that DRIL is a dynamic phenomenon. Its reversibility, with an anatomic improvement, decreases with increasing duration [58, 68]. Thus, DRIL seems to be a biomarker that may be incorporated into daily clinical practice and be a useful tool in the future therapeutic intervention [69].

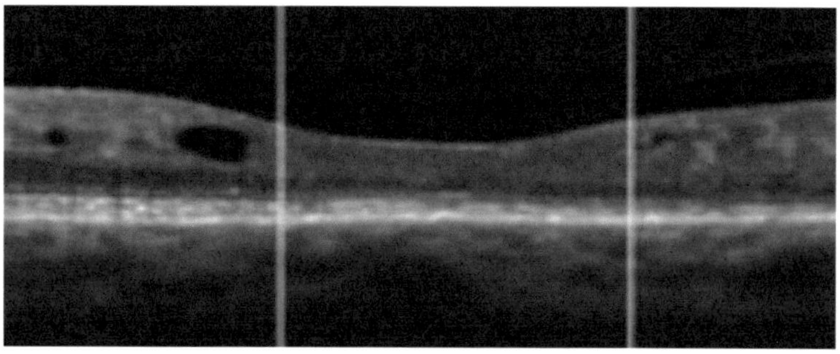

Figure 9.
DRIL areas in SD-OCT.

3.8 Pearl necklace sign

The pearl necklace sign refers to HRD in a continuous ring around the cystoid spaces in the retina that has been seen in diseases with exudative maculopathy, vascular leakage, and chronic CME such as neovascular AMD, DME, retinal vein occlusion, retinal arterial macroaneurysm, or Coats disease (**Figure 10**) [70]. The authors speculated that HRD indicated the presence of lipid material from retinal vascular leakage similar to hard exudates. These pearls may represent lipid-filled macrophages along the inner wall of retinal edema [70]. Moreover, it is considered a frequent precursor sign on the location of the hard exudates which appear later. Therefore, this sign can change shape and may resolve under treatment or spontaneously. The presence of pearl necklace sign has not been associated with worse visual acuity in RD [71].

The pearl necklace sign should be differentiated from ORTs, which are located deeper in the ONL of the retina. In ORT, the ring is continuous and homogeneous, whereas the hyperreflective ring is as small foci in the pearl necklace sign [3].

3.9 Focal choroidal excavation (FCE)

FCE is a localized depression of the choroid detected only by using OCT, without any evidence of posterior staphyloma or scleral ectasia. It affects Bruch's membrane-RPE-choriocapillaris line complex line and photoreceptors (**Figure 11**). Patients are mostly asymptomatic and have good visual acuity. Nevertheless, some lesions may be associated with the development of choroidal neovascular membrane. It has been reported that FCE may appear in certain macular disorders such as CSCR, AMD, ERM, CNVM, polypoidal choroidal vasculopathy, BVMD, Vogt-Koyanagi-Harada disease, punctate inner choroidopathy, focal retinochoroiditis, foveoschisis, torpedo maculopathy, multiple evanescent white dot syndrome, multifocal choroiditis, and combined hamartoma of the retina and RPE [3]. OCT allows to identify retinal and choroidal structures that are affected in the excavation, which usually includes RPE, Bruch's membrane, EZ line, ELM, and ONL which followed the contour of the FCE. In some cases, it can be appreciated an attenuation or absence of IS/OS junction at the excavation, and ONL was thickened in most conforming eyes [72]. However, the layers from the OPL to the ILM were undisturbed, and also the sclerochoroidal junction appeared reasonably preserved without scleral excavation [72, 73]. FCE may be organized in two patterns, whether or not the photoreceptor layer is detached

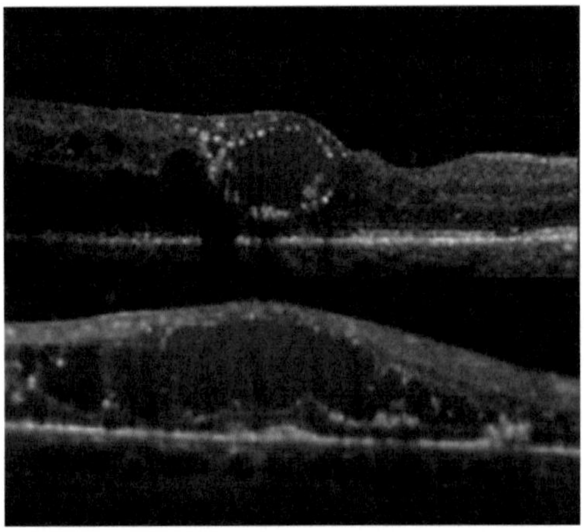

Figure 10.
Pearl necklace sign in patients with severe diabetic macular edema.

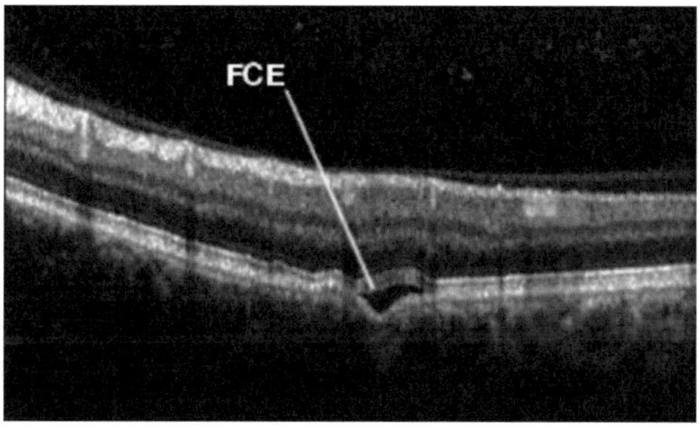

Figure 11.
Focal choroidal excavation (FCE) revealed by SD-OCT in a patient with chronic CSCR and systemic lupus erythematosus.

from the RPE. Thus, conforming FCE describes those types of lesions without separation between the two layers and the photoreceptors adapt to the contour of the RPE layer. On the other hand, in nonconforming FCE, photoreceptors appeared to be detached from the RPE showing a hyporeflective space. Factors contributing to the formation of each pattern are unknown [74]. Other authors have classified the lesions into three morphological patterns based on SD-OCT findings: bowl shaped, cone shaped, and mixed shaped [75]. They observed that all bowl-shaped types showed atrophic changes and RPE irregularities, whereas in cone-shaped FCE, a less atrophic change is detected at the center of the lesion. The pathogenesis of FCE is still unknown. Some authors suggest it could be related to a congenital defect within the choroid, which is supported by the fact that shape and size remained stable during the follow-up in most of the reported cases [73]. Nevertheless, no family history and low prevalence in young people suggest that it may be an acquired condition [74]. Some authors proposed FCE is an entity related to inflammatory diseases like Vogt-Koyanagi-Harada disease, multiple evanescent white dot syndrome, and other types of retinochoroiditis [76].

3.10 Foveal pseudocyst

Foveal pseudocyst is an OCT pathologic sign that is caused by subretinal retention of perfluorocarbon liquid (PFCL) after vitreoretinal surgery. Subretinal PFCL is a serious complication if it affects fovea. The incidence ranges from 1 to 11% after retinal detachment surgery [77]. Main risk factors for this entity are the presence of a large size retinal tear, large retinotomy (especially in 360°), and retinal traction at retinal breaks [78]. It is rare to find it in conventional surgery, but in these cases, it is usually caused by small bubbles which can be produced by turbulence by the interface between PFCL and saline solution [77]. OCT is a useful tool to identify intraretinal bubbles of PFCL. In many cases, the bubbles remain stable without size changing. The most common signs in OCT are RPE pigment disorganization, disruption of ellipsoid layer, and hyperreflectivity at the base of the PFCL bubble (**Figure 12**) [77]. It has been reported several cases with retinal hole secondary to long-standing subretinal PFCL [79]. Subretinal PFCL is responsible for retinal damage resulting in loss of visual acuity, scotomas, and retinal thinning. Long-time exposure to PFCL can lead to RPE atrophy, photoreceptor damage because there is a direct toxic defect, or inflammatory response including macrophages phagocyted PFCL [77]. It is recommended to remove PFCL bubbles located beneath the macula or if there is a tendency to move to the macular area [80].

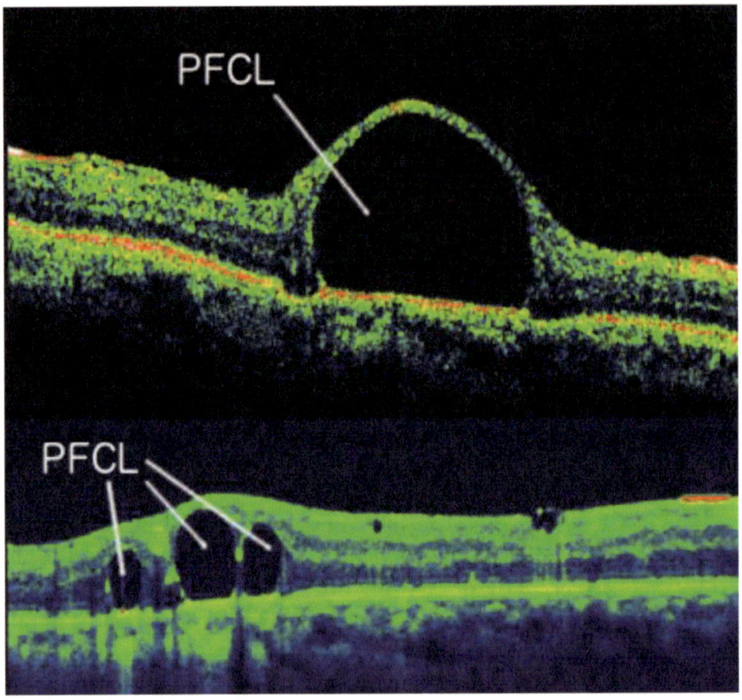

Figure 12.
Subretinal retention of perfluorocarbon liquid (PFCL) after retinal detachment surgery.

3.11 Choroidal macrovessel

It is a rare ocular lesion which appears on fundus examination as an abnormal, tortuous vessel deep to the retina. It was first described as a serpiginoid atrophic lesion in the temporal macula, with an orange-red aspect and several unspecific choroidal spots in the posterior pole [81]. Choroidal macrovessel is not associated with acute inflammation and symptoms. Some reports have shown hyperpigmentation of the RPE, debris in the subretinal space, and changes in the outer nuclear layer (ONL) thickness [82, 83]. SD-OCT reveals a tubular structure which shows hyperreflectivity band below RPE representing the superior edge of the lesion, with an elevation of RPE and photoreceptor and posterior shadowing [81]. In recent studies, it has been explored with enhanced-depth imaging spectral domain optical coherence tomography (EDI SD-OCT) showing a vascular structure that traversed the entire choroidal thickness and produces an indentation at the choroidal-scleral junction and the ellipsoid zone (EZ) causing a reduction of the ONL thickness [82, 83]. A differential diagnosis from choroidal macrovessel should be made with subretinal nematode tract, choroidal hemangioma, inflammatory choroidopathy, retinochoroidal anastomosis, vortex varix, and aberrant long posterior ciliary artery [81, 83].

3.12 Dipping sign

It is a pathologic retinal sign that may be appreciated with high-resolution OCT images in some patients with acute CSCR. It is characterized by getting an inverted triangle shape at the outer surface of the detached retina, in those eyes with fibrinous exudate in the subretinal space that protrudes over the RPE [3]. The primary cause of dipping sign seems to be traction due to the fibrinous exudates and the swelling of the ONL. It has been reported that some of the leakage sites (20.3%) show fibrinous exudate as a highly reflective area in the subretinal space, around the leakage site [84]. Additional observations with SD-OCT include thickening of the outer photoreceptor segment layer with invisibility of the inner segment-outer segment junction line and "dipping" of the posterior retinal layer toward the RPE [84, 85]. In later stages, granular deposits may become visible at the posterior surface of the detached retina [85]. It has been documented a decrease in foveal thickness once CSCR is resolved.

3.13 Cystoid foveal degeneration (CDF)

CDF is a rare form of macular pathology that can be precisely diagnosed only with OCT. It is characterized by large cystic spaces, or in some cases, giant single cyst in the fovea. It can occur with or without thinned septa between cystic spaces. Usually, it affects patients with diabetic maculopathy, uveitis, RVO, AMD, associated with Streptococcus constellatus endocarditis, and CSR [3, 86]. The hyperreflective OCT appearance of these lesions, followed by cystic change and permanent visual loss, suggests that they might represent retinal infarctions. Their predilection for the fovea may reflect the high metabolic demand at this area of the retina and the narrow-bore capillaries of the perifoveal vasculature.

This pathology is associated with a distortion of IS/OS layer and loss of outer segment of photoreceptors. In comparison with CME, CDF has a more extensive and multitude cysts. As opposed to CME, although CDF cysts may shrink or disappear, there is a limited improvement in visual acuity [3]. FA and fundus autofluorescence (FAF) are not capable of distinguishing CME from CDF.

Acknowledgements

Thanks to Antonio Arias Palomero and José Juan Valdés González for the effort of searching some of the images showed in this chapter.

Conflicts of interest

Dr. Ascaso reports nonfinancial support from Topcon and Zeiss. All remaining authors have declared no conflicts of interest. All coauthors have seen and agreed with the contents of the manuscript.

Author details

Francisco Javier Lara-Medina[1,2*], Olivia Esteban[1,2], Isabel Bartolomé[1,2], C. Ispa[1,2], Javier Mateo[1,2] and Francisco Javier Ascaso[1,2,3]

1 Department of Ophthalmology, Hospital Clínico Universitario "Lozano Blesa", Zaragoza, Spain

2 Aragon Health Research Institute (IIS Aragon), Zaragoza, Spain

3 School of Medicine, University of Zaragoza, Zaragoza, Spain

*Address all correspondence to: javierlara@me.com

References

[1] Arevalo JF, Lasave AF, Arias J, Serrano M, Arevalo F. Clinical applications of optical coherence tomography in the posterior pole: The 2011 José Manuel Espino lecture—part I. Clinical Ophthalmology. 2013;7:2165-2179

[2] Chauhan DS, Antcliff RJ, Rai PA, Williamson TH, Marshall J. Papillofoveal traction in macular hole formation: The role of optical coherence tomography. Archives of Ophthalmology. 2000;**118**(1):32-38

[3] Turgut B, Demir T. The new landmarks, findings and signs in optical coherence tomography. New Frontiers in Ophthalmology. 2016;**2**(3):131-136

[4] Staurenghi G, Sadda S, Chakravarthy U, Spaide RF. Proposed lexicon for anatomic landmarks in normal posterior segment spectral-domain optical coherence tomography. Ophthalmology. 2014;**121**(8):1572-1578

[5] Saxena S, Srivastav K, Cheung CM, Ng JY, Lai TY. Photoreceptor inner segment ellipsoid band integrity on spectral domain optical coherence tomography. Clinical Ophthalmology. 2014;**8**:2507-2522

[6] Spaide RF, Curcio CA. Anatomical correlates to the bands seen in the outer retina by optical coherence tomography: Literature review and model. Retina. 2011;**31**(8):1609-1619

[7] Mitamura Y, Mitamura-Aizawa S, Katome T, Naito T, Hagiwara A, Kumagai K, et al. Photoreceptor impairment and restoration on optical coherence tomographic image. Journal of Ophthalmology. 2013;**2013**:1-7

[8] Aizawa S, Mitamura Y, Hagiwara A, Sugawara T, Yamamoto S. Changes of fundus autofluorescence, photoreceptor inner and outer segment junction line, and visual function in patients with retinitis pigmentosa: Autofluorescence in retinitis pigmentosa. Clinical & Experimental Ophthalmology. 2010;**38**(6):597-604

[9] Wakabayashi T, Oshima Y, Fujimoto H, Murakami Y, Sakaguchi H, Kusaka S, et al. Foveal microstructure and visual acuity after retinal detachment repair. Ophthalmology. 2009;**116**(3):519-528

[10] Bottoni F, De Angelis S, Luccarelli S, Cigada M, Staurenghi G. The dynamic healing process of idiopathic macular holes after surgical repair: A spectral-domain optical coherence tomography study. Investigative Ophthalmology & Visual Science. 2011;**52**(7):4439

[11] Ooka E, Mitamura Y, Baba T, Kitahashi M, Oshitari T, Yamamoto S. Foveal microstructure on spectral-domain optical coherence tomographic images and visual function after macular hole surgery. American Journal of Ophthalmology. 2011;**152**(2): 283-290.e1

[12] Shimozono M, Oishi A, Hata M, Kurimoto Y. Restoration of the photoreceptor outer segment and visual outcomes after macular hole closure: Spectral-domain optical coherence tomography analysis. Graefe's Archive for Clinical and Experimental Ophthalmology. 2011;**249**(10):1469-1476

[13] Wakabayashi T, Fujiwara M, Sakaguchi H, Kusaka S, Oshima Y. Foveal microstructure and visual acuity in surgically closed macular holes: Spectral-domain optical coherence tomographic analysis. Ophthalmology. 2010;**117**(9):1815-1824

[14] Oishi A, Shimozono M, Mandai M, Hata M, Nishida A, Kurimoto Y. Recovery of photoreceptor outer segments after anti-VEGF therapy for

age-related macular degeneration. Graefe's Archive for Clinical and Experimental Ophthalmology. 2013;**251**(2):435-440

[15] Hartmann KI, Gomez ML, Bartsch D-UG, Schuster AK, Freeman WR. Effect of change in drusen evolution on photoreceptor inner segment/outer segment junction. Retina. 2012;**32**(8):1492-1499

[16] Mrejen S, Sato T, Curcio CA, Spaide RF. Assessing the cone photoreceptor mosaic in eyes with pseudodrusen and soft drusen in vivo using adaptive optics imaging. Ophthalmology. 2014;**121**(2):545-551

[17] Curcio CA, Messinger JD, Sloan KR, McGwin G, Medeiros NE, Spaide RF. Subretinal drusenoid deposits in non-neovascular age-related macular degeneration: Morphology, prevalence, topography, and biogenesis model. Retina. 2013;**33**(2):265-276

[18] Pilotto E, Benetti E, Convento E, Guidolin F, Longhin E, Parrozzani R, et al. Microperimetry, fundus autofluorescence, and retinal layer changes in progressing geographic atrophy. Canadian Journal of Ophthalmology. 2013;**48**(5):386-393

[19] Maheshwary AS, Oster SF, Yuson RMS, Cheng L, Mojana F, Freeman WR. The association between percent disruption of the photoreceptor inner segment-outer segment junction and visual acuity in diabetic macular edema. American Journal of Ophthalmology. 2010;**150**(1):63-67.e1

[20] Jain A, Saxena S, Khanna VK, Shukla RK, Meyer CH. Status of serum VEGF and ICAM-1 and its association with external limiting membrane and inner segment-outer segment junction disruption in type 2 diabetes mellitus. Molecular Vision. 2013;**19**:1760-1768

[21] Itoh Y, Inoue M, Rii T, Hirota K, Hirakata A. Correlation between foveal cone outer segment tips line and visual recovery after epiretinal membrane surgery. Investigative Ophthalmology & Visual Science. 2013;**54**(12):7302

[22] Inoue M, Morita S, Watanabe Y, Kaneko T, Yamane S, Kobayashi S, et al. Inner segment/outer segment junction assessed by spectral-domain optical coherence tomography in patients with idiopathic epiretinal membrane. American Journal of Ophthalmology. 2010;**150**(6):834-839

[23] Suh MH, Seo JM, Park KH, Yu HG. Associations between macular findings by optical coherence tomography and visual outcomes after epiretinal membrane removal. American Journal of Ophthalmology. 2009;**147**(3):473-480.e3

[24] Gharbiya M, Grandinetti F, Scavella V, Cecere M, Esposito M, Segnalini A, et al. Correlation between spectral-domain optical coherence tomography findings and visual outcome after primary rhegmatogenous retinal detachment repair. Retina. 2012;**32**(1):43-53

[25] Coscas G, De Benedetto U, Coscas F, Li Calzi CI, Vismara S, Roudot-Thoraval F, et al. Hyperreflective dots: A new spectral-domain optical coherence tomography entity for follow-up and prognosis in exudative age-related macular degeneration. Ophthalmologica. 2013;**229**(1):32-37

[26] Bolz M, Schmidt-Erfurth U, Deak G, Mylonas G, Kriechbaum K, Scholda C. Optical coherence tomographic hyperreflective foci. Ophthalmology. 2009;**116**(5):914-920

[27] Vujosevic S, Bini S, Midena G, Berton M, Pilotto E, Midena E. Hyperreflective intraretinal spots in diabetics without and with nonproliferative diabetic retinopathy: An in vivo study using spectral domain OCT. Journal Diabetes Research. 2013;**2013**:1-5

[28] Vujosevic S, Torresin T, Bini S, Convento E, Pilotto E, Parrozzani R, et al. Imaging retinal inflammatory biomarkers after intravitreal steroid and anti-VEGF treatment in diabetic macular oedema. Acta Ophthalmologica. 2017;**95**(5):464-471

[29] Coscas G, Loewenstein A, Augustin A, Bandello F, Battaglia Parodi M, Lanzetta P, et al. Management of retinal vein occlusion—Consensus document. Ophthalmologica. 2011;**226**(1):4-28

[30] Ogino K, Murakami T, Tsujikawa A, Miyamoto K, Sakamoto A, Ota M, et al. Characteristics of optical coherence tomographic hyperreflective foci in retinal vein occlusion. Retina. 2012;**32**(1):77-85

[31] Uji A, Murakami T, Nishijima K, Akagi T, Horii T, Arakawa N, et al. Association between hyperreflective foci in the outer retina, status of photoreceptor layer, and visual acuity in diabetic macular edema. American Journal of Ophthalmology. 2012;**153**(4):710-717.e1

[32] Hwang HS, Chae JB, Kim JY, Kim DY. Association between hyperreflective dots on spectral-domain optical coherence tomography in macular edema and response to treatment. Investigative Ophthalmology & Visual Science. 2017;**58**(13):5958

[33] Mavrikakis I, Sfikakis PP, Mavrikakis E, Rougas K, Nikolaou A, Kostopoulos C, et al. The incidence of irreversible retinal toxicity in patients treated with hydroxychloroquine: A reappraisal. Ophthalmology. 2003;**110**(7):1321-1326

[34] Chen E, Brown DM, Benz MS, Fish RH, Wong TP, Kim RY, et al. Spectral domain optical coherence tomography as an effective screening test for hydroxychloroquine retinopathy (the "flying saucer" sign). Clinical Ophthalmology. 2010;**4**:1151-1158

[35] Ascaso FJ, Rodríguez NA, San Miguel R, Huerva V. The "flying saucer" sign on spectral domain optical coherence tomography in chloroquine retinopathy. Arthritis and Rheumatism. 2013;**65**(9):2322-2322

[36] Zweifel SA. Outer retinal tubulation: A novel optical coherence tomography finding. Archives of Ophthalmology. 2009;**127**(12):1596

[37] Iriyama A, Aihara Y, Yanagi Y. Outer retinal tubulation in inherited retinal degenerative disease. Retina. 2013;**33**(7):1462-1465

[38] Goldberg NR, Greenberg JP, Laud K, Tsang S, Freund KB. Outer retinal tubbulation in degeneration retinal disorders. Retina. 2013;**33**(9):1871-1876

[39] Zweifel SA, Imamura Y, Freund KB, Spaide RF. Multimodal fundus imaging of pseudoxanthoma elasticum. Retina. 2011;**31**(3):482-491

[40] Sambricio J, Tejada-Palacios P, Barceló-Mendiguchía A. Choroidal neovascularization, outer retinal tubulation and fundus autofluorescence findings in a patient with enhanced S-cone syndrome. Clinical & Experimental Ophthalmology. 2016;**44**(1):69-71

[41] Schaal KB, Freund KB, Litts KM, Zhang Y, Messinger JD, Curcio CA. Outer retinal tubulation in advanced age-related macular degeneration: Optical coherence tomographic findings correspond to histology. Retina. 2015;**35**(7):1339-1350

[42] Dolz-Marco R, Litts KM, Tan ACS, Freund KB, Curcio CA. The evolution of outer retinal tubulation, a neurodegeneration and gliosis prominent in macular diseases. Ophthalmology. 2017;**124**(9):1353-1367

[43] Caillaux V, Gaucher D, Gualino V, Massin P, Tadayoni R, Gaudric A.

Morphologic characterization of dome-shaped macula in myopic eyes with serous macular detachment. American Journal of Ophthalmology. 2013;**156**(5):958-967.e1

[44] Errera M-H, Michaelides M, Keane PA, Restori M, Paques M, Moore AT, et al. The extended clinical phenotype of dome-shaped macula. Graefe's Archive for Clinical and Experimental Ophthalmology. 2014;**252**(3):499-508

[45] Keane PA, Mitra A, Khan IJ, Quhill F, Elsherbiny SM. Dome-shaped macula: A compensatory mechanism in myopic anisometropia? Ophthalmic Surgery, Lasers & Imaging: The Official Journal of the International Society for Imaging in the Eye. 2012;**43 Online**:e52-e54

[46] Imamura Y, Iida T, Maruko I, Zweifel SA, Spaide RF. Enhanced depth imaging optical coherence tomography of the sclera in dome-shaped macula. American Journal of Ophthalmology. 2011;**151**(2):297-302

[47] Mehdizadeh M, Nowroozzadeh MH. Dome-shaped macula in eyes with myopic posterior staphyloma. American Journal of Ophthalmology. 2008;**146**(3):478-479

[48] Gaucher D, Erginay A, Lecleire-Collet A, Haouchine B, Puech M, Cohen S-Y, et al. Dome-shaped macula in eyes with myopic posterior staphyloma. American Journal of Ophthalmology. 2008;**145**(5):909-914

[49] Ellabban AA, Tsujikawa A, Matsumoto A, Yamashiro K, Oishi A, Ooto S, et al. Three-dimensional tomographic features of dome-shaped macula by swept-source optical coherence tomography. American Journal of Ophthalmology. 2013;**155**(2):320-328.e2

[50] Ohsugi H, Ikuno Y, Oshima K, Yamauchi T, Tabuchi H. Morphologic characteristics of macular complications of a dome-shaped macula determined by swept-source optical coherence tomography. American Journal of Ophthalmology. 2014;**158**(1):162-170.e1

[51] Lorenzo D, Arias L, Choudhry N, Millan E, Flores I, Rubio MJ, et al. Dome-shaped macula in myopic eyes: Twelve-month follow-up. Retina. 2017;**37**(4):680-686

[52] Soudier G, Gaudric A, Gualino V, Massin P, Nardin M, Tadayoni R, et al. Long-term evolution of dome-shaped macula: Increased macular bulge is associated with extended macular atrophy. Retina. 2016;**36**(5):944-952

[53] Daruich A, Matet A, Dirani A, Bousquet E, Zhao M, Farman N, et al. Central serous chorioretinopathy: Recent findings and new physiopathology hypothesis. Progress in Retinal and Eye Research. 2015;**48**:82-118

[54] Matsumoto H, Kishi S, Sato T, Mukai R. Fundus autofluorescence of elongated photoreceptor outer segments in central serous chorioretinopathy. American Journal of Ophthalmology. 2011;**151**(4):617-623.e1

[55] Spaide RF, Klancnik JM. Fundus autofluorescence and central serous chorioretinopathy. Ophthalmology. 2005;**112**(5):825-833

[56] Drexler W, Morgner U, Ghanta RK, Kärtner FX, Schuman JS, Fujimoto JG. Ultrahigh-resolution ophthalmic optical coherence tomography. Nature Medicine. 2001;7(4):502-507

[57] Pianta MJ, Aleman TS, Cideciyan AV, Sunness JS, Li Y, Campochiaro BA, et al. In vivo micropathology of best macular dystrophy with optical coherence tomography. Experimental Eye Research. 2003;**76**(2):203-211

[58] Sun JK, Radwan SH, Soliman AZ, Lammer J, Lin MM, Prager SG, et al.

Neural retinal disorganization as a robust marker of visual acuity in current and resolved diabetic macular edema. Diabetes. 2015;**64**(7):2560-2570

[59] Nicholson L, Ramu J, Triantafyllopoulou I, Patrao NV, Comyn O, Hykin P, et al. Diagnostic accuracy of disorganization of the retinal inner layers in detecting macular capillary non-perfusion in diabetic retinopathy. Clinical & Experimental Ophthalmology. 2015;**43**(8):735-741

[60] Moein H-R, Novais EA, Rebhun CB, Cole ED, Louzada RN, Witkin AJ, et al. Optical coherence tomography angiography to detect macular capillary ischemia in patients with inner retinal changes after resolved diabetic macular edema. Retina. 2018;**38**(12):2277-2284

[61] Bek T. Transretinal histopathological changes in capillary-free areas of diabetic retinopathy. Acta Ophthalmologica. 1994; **72**(4):409-415

[62] Barber AJ, Lieth E, Khin SA, Antonetti DA, Buchanan AG, Gardner TW. Neural apoptosis in the retina during experimental and human diabetes. Early onset and effect of insulin. The Journal of Clinical Investigation. 1998;**102**(4):783-791

[63] Grewal DS, O'Sullivan ML, Kron M, Jaffe GJ. Association of disorganization of retinal inner layers with visual acuity in eyes with uveitic cystoid macular edema. American Journal of Ophthalmology. 2017;**177**:116-125

[64] Berry D, Thomas AS, Fekrat S, Grewal DS. Association of disorganization of retinal inner layers with ischemic index and visual acuity in central retinal vein occlusion. Ophthalmology Retina. 2018;**2**(11):1125-1132

[65] Balaratnasingam C, Inoue M, Ahn S, McCann J, Dhrami-Gavazi E, Yannuzzi LA, et al. Visual acuity is correlated with the area of the foveal avascular zone in diabetic retinopathy and retinal vein occlusion. Ophthalmology. 2016;**123**(11):2352-2367

[66] Joltikov KA, Sesi CA, de Castro VM, Davila JR, Anand R, Khan SM, et al. Disorganization of retinal inner layers (DRIL) and neuroretinal dysfunction in early diabetic retinopathy. Investigative Ophthalmology & Visual Science. 2018;**59**(13):5481-5486

[67] Das R, Spence G, Hogg RE, Stevenson M, Chakravarthy U. Disorganization of inner retina and outer retinal morphology in diabetic macular edema. JAMA Ophthalmology. 2018;**136**(2):202-208

[68] Radwan SH, Soliman AZ, Tokarev J, Zhang L, van Kuijk FJ, Koozekanani DD. Association of disorganization of retinal inner layers with vision after resolution of center-involved diabetic macular edema. JAMA Ophthalmology. 2015;**133**(7):820-825

[69] Sun JK, Lin MM, Lammer J, Prager S, Sarangi R, Silva PS, et al. Disorganization of the retinal inner layers as a predictor of visual acuity in eyes with center-involved diabetic macular edema. JAMA Ophthalmology. 2014;**132**(11):1309-1316

[70] Gelman SK, Freund KB, Shah VP, Sarraf D. The pearl necklace sign: A novel spectral domain optical coherence tomography finding in exudative macular disease. Retina. 2014;**34**(10):2088-2095

[71] Ajay K, Mason F, Gonglore B, Bhatnagar A. Pearl necklace sign in diabetic macular edema: Evaluation and significance. Indian Journal of Ophthalmology. 2016;**64**(11):829-834

[72] Liu G-H, Lin B, Sun X-Q, He Z-F, Li J-R, Zhou R, et al. Focal choroidal excavation: A preliminary interpretation based on clinic and review. International

Journal of Ophthalmology. 2015;**8**(3):513-521

[73] Lee CS, Woo SJ, Kim Y-K, Hwang DJ, Kang HM, Kim H, et al. Clinical and spectral-domain optical coherence tomography findings in patients with focal choroidal excavation. Ophthalmology. 2014;**121**(5):1029-1035

[74] Chung CY, Li SH, Li KKW. Focal choroidal excavation-morphological features and clinical correlation. Eye. 2017;**31**(9):1373-1379

[75] Shinojima A, Kawamura A, Mori R, Yuzawa M. Morphologic features of focal choroidal excavation on spectral domain optical coherence tomography with simultaneous angiography. Retina. 2014;**34**(7):1407-1414

[76] Hashimoto Y, Saito W, Noda K, Ishida S. Acquired focal choroidal excavation associated with multiple evanescent white dot syndrome: Observations at onset and a pathogenic hypothesis. BMC Ophthalmology. 2014;**14**(1):135

[77] Liu W, Gao M, Liang X. Management of subfoveal perfluorocarbon liquid: A review. Ophthalmologica. 2018;**240**(1):1-7

[78] Garcia-Valenzuela E, Ito Y, Abrams GW. Risk factors for retention of subretinal perfluorocarbon liquid in vitreoretinal surgery. Retina. 2004;**24**(5):746-752

[79] Cohen SY, Dubois L, Elmaleh C. Retinal hole as a complication of long-standing subretinal perfluorocarbon liquid. Retina. 2006;**26**(7):843-844

[80] Roth DB, Sears JE, Lewis H. Removal of retained subfoveal perfluoro-n-octane liquid. American Journal of Ophthalmology. 2004;**138**(2):287-289

[81] Lima LH, Laud K, Chang LK, Yannuzzi LA. Choroidal macrovessel. The British Journal of Ophthalmology. 2011;**95**(9):1333-1334

[82] Ehlers JP, Rayess H, Spaide RF. Isolated choroidal macrovessel: A tracklike choroidal lesion. Canadian Journal of Ophthalmology. 2014;**49**(6):e158-e160

[83] Choudhry N, Rao RC. Enhanced depth imaging features of a choroidal macrovessel. Retinal Cases and Brief Reports. 2016;**10**(1):18-21

[84] Kim HC, Cho WB, Chung H. Morphologic changes in acute central serous chorioretinopathy using spectral domain optical coherence tomography. Korean Journal of Ophthalmology. 2012;**26**(5):347-354

[85] Fujimoto H, Gomi F, Wakabayashi T, Sawa M, Tsujikawa M, Tano Y. Morphologic changes in acute central serous chorioretinopathy evaluated by Fourier-domain optical coherence tomography. Ophthalmology. 2008;**115**(9):1494-1500.e2

[86] Thaisiam P, Rattanaumpawan P. Rare manifestations of Streptococcus pneumoniae infection; the first case report in Thailand and literature review of pneumococcal endophthalmitis and endocarditis. Journal of the Medical Association of Thailand. 2014;**97**(12):1364-1369

Chapter 6

Swept-Source Optical Coherence Tomography and Optical Coherence Tomography Angiography in Selected Posterior Uveitides

Magdy Moussa and Mahmoud Leila

Abstract

The pathogenesis of uveitis entails changes in the structural morphology of the macula, choroid, and choroidal perfusion. Documentation of these pathologic alterations is pivotal in making a proper diagnosis and in follow-up of outcomes of therapy. The newly-introduced swept-source optical coherence tomography (SS-OCT) and optical coherence tomography angiography (SS-OCTA) were harbingers of a whole new era of noninvasive in vivo layer-to-layer dissection of macular and choroidal structural changes in uveitis and of disease-related vascular profile patterns. This new information unraveled new aspects of the underlying pathogenetic mechanisms in different uveitides and added to our understanding of the disease process. Monitoring choroidal thickness was introduced as a novel sensitive index for evaluation and titration of treatment response. Moreover, the ensuing complications of uveitis as poor pupillary dilatation due to posterior synechiae and mild to moderate opacities due to cataract or vitritis that frequently posed pertinacious impediments for reproducible imaging were overcome by SS-OCT features notably long-wavelength scanning laser and reduced sensitivity roll-off features. In the current manuscript we present our experience in diagnosis and management of selected posterior uveitides using SS-OCT and SS-OCTA.

Keywords: swept-source OCT in uveitis, swept-source OCTA in uveitis, Vogt-Koyanagi-Harada, serpiginous choroiditis, multifocal choroiditis, punctate inner choroidopathy, toxoplasmosis

1. Introduction

Traditionally, management of posterior segment inflammation secondary to uveitis relied on fundus fluorescein angiography (FFA) and indocyanine green angiography (ICG) for assessment of the pathological alteration of the inner- and outer-blood-retina-barriers (BRB), disturbances in choroidal perfusion, and the structural sequelae of inflammation in the macular area and elsewhere in the retina and the choroid [1, 2]. These tests offered indirect biological clues to evaluate the quality of the retinal and choroidal circulations in terms of patterns of leakage and grades of perfusion; henceforth, determination of disease evolution through remissions and exacerbations, titration of posology and monitoring tissue response to therapy [3, 4].

1.1 Limitations of conventional angiographic modalities

Despite the invaluable input of these diagnostic tools, they had inherent limitations that posed major impediment to full exploration of the pathological events in the posterior segment secondary to different uveitides. Firstly, the profuse leakage of the sodium fluorescein molecule from the choriocapillaris, and the optical scattering of incident light by the retinal nerve fiber layer confined the utility of FFA mostly to single-layered evaluation of the pathological cascade of events developing at the level of superficial capillary plexus (SCP) and left the observer with vague deductions regarding the ongoing pathology in the deep capillary plexus (DCP), the choriocapillaris and the choroidal stroma [5–9]. Secondly, the inflammatory by-products of uveitides and the associated pathological features included intra-, sub-retinal and sub-retinal pigment epithelium (RPE) fluid and/or lipoproteinaceous deposits, sub-retinal and sub-RPE fibrosis, RPE thickening and pigment epithelial detachment (PED). These features shared common FFA leakage and ICG fluorescence properties among themselves and with choroidal neovascular membrane (CNV) that might complicate posterior segment inflammation, which made these entities virtually indistinguishable from each other and subsequently delayed diagnosis and prompt intervention for treating CNV. Thirdly, the longevity of uveitis disease process and its propensity to undulating course of remissions and exacerbations render repetitive dye-based FFA and ICG angiography impractical and even hazardous in routine clinical practice due to their invasive nature [3, 4, 10].

1.2 Swept-source optical coherence tomography (SS-OCT) and optical coherence tomography angiography (SS-OCTA) technology: novel imaging modality in uveitides

The introduction of swept-source optical coherence tomography (SS-OCT) technology revolutionized imaging of ocular posterior segment in uveitides and circumvented several classical obstacles that long represented significant hindrance to correct diagnosis. Firstly, SS-OCT employed a long wavelength laser source (1050 nm) operating at an ultra-high scanning speed (100.000 A-scan/second). The tandem of ultra-high-speed image acquisition, laser beam collimation and reduced sensitivity roll-off feature helped defraying scattering of the scanning light as it traveled through the retina, with subsequent rendition of ultra-high-definition images of retinal layers quasi-in-vivo histological tissue dissection [11, 12]

Moreover, these features enhanced beam penetration in media opacities and poorly dilatable pupils, which are common features associated with uveitis and that pose significant impediment to interpretable images. New morphological changes in the vitreo-retinal interface, the retina, the choroidal layers, and changes in choroidal thickness secondary to uveitides were unveiled and employed as biomarkers for diagnosis of uveitis, detection of ensuing complications and monitoring disease progression and response to therapy. Secondly, superior axial resolution and greater depth of penetration of the incident beam in enhanced depth (EDI)- and SS-OCT imaging allowed simultaneous documentation of pathological changes in the vitreous, vitreo-retinal interface, retina, and choroid in a single frame amenable to scrutiny and exploration of the true magnitude of tissue involvement by the disease process [13–18].

Thirdly, SS-OCT incorporated a blood flow detection algorithm; OCTARA (Optical Coherence Tomography Angiography Ratio Analysis). This novel feature allowed evaluation of the retinal vascular plexuses and of the choriocapillaris that are frequently targeted in uveitides. The algorithm relies on decorrelation motion contrast between rapidly repeated SS-OCT B-scans to visualize blood flow in vivo without the need for contrast injection. This OCTA implement benefits from being merged with SS-OCT technology to generate separate en-face images of the retinal SCP, DCP, and the choriocapillaris. It is worthy of note that OCTARA algorithm generates OCTA images by registering B-scan repetition at each scan location then computing a ratio-based result between corresponding image pixels. This method preserves the integrity of the OCT spectrum and does not result in compromised axial resolution, an inherent disadvantage of other OCTA technologies [19–22].

OCTA excelled in delineating inflammatory CNV that could complicate posterior uveitis and determining its state whether active, quiescent, or recurrent based on the neovascular network morphological criteria [10, 23, 24]. Inflammatory CNV has long posed a diagnostic predicament in the past due to overlapping leakage and/or fluorescence patterns with non-neovascular inflammatory tissue on FFA and ICG, respectively. Likewise, CNV and non-neovascular inflammatory lesions frequently exhibit similar light backscattering properties that render them indistinguishable from each other on structural OCT [3, 4, 25, 26].

It is worthy of note that OCTA does not provide information on vascular leakage, which is a crucial index of the integrity of the inner BRB in cases of vasculitis associated with uveitides. In cases of active vasculitis, OCTA could be even misleading as the leakage of plasma from a disrupted inner BRB into the extra-cellular compartment might slow-down the blood stream velocity well below the detection threshold of OCTA, which might be falsely interpreted by OCTA as reduced vessel density and capillary non-perfusion [3].

2. Authors' case presentations

In the following case presentations, we present our experience with SS-OCT and SS-OCTA using the swept-source DRI OCT Triton machine version 10.11 (Topcon Corporation, Tokyo, Japan) and the OCTARA algorithm (Topcon Corporation, Tokyo, Japan), respectively, in imaging common non-infectious and infectious uveitides, with emphasis on the importance of multi-modal imaging approach in which different imaging modalities complement one another to reveal the true extent of the ongoing pathology.

2.1 Non-infectious uveitides

2.1.1 Vogt-Koyanagi-Harada (VKH)

VKH is a multi-system disorder featuring ocular, auditory, integumentary, and neurological manifestations. Ocular involvement in VKH is in the form of bilateral granulomatous panuveitis that is notorious of profound drop of vision, hence the need for early aggressive treatment. Posterior segment involvement in the acute stage comprises diffuse choroiditis, optic disc hyperemia, multifocal serous retinal detachment or bullous exudative retinal detachment. As the chronic stage of the disease ensues, the patient develops ocular depigmentation in the form of chorioretinal depigmented scars and retinal pigmentary disturbances [27, 28].

The primary target tissue in VKH is the choroidal stroma which endures dense infiltration with inflammatory cells and subsequent thickening due to engorgement of choroidal vessels and serous exudation. Eventually, the RPE dehisces giving way to the inflammatory infiltrates and serous fluid into the sub-retinal space. RPE folds develop due to displacement by the thickened choroid. The choriocapillaris undergoes ischemic changes especially in recurrent cases in the form of localized vascular loss. This could be explained by severe hypoperfusion secondary to inflammation or by pressure atrophy from inflammatory granulomas

[29, 30]. These areas of choriocapillaris loss appear on OCTA examination as sharply demarcated flow-voids that might recover after resolution of inflammation [31, 32]. Recurrent attacks of inflammation with subsequent breaching of the RPE-Bruch's complex could trigger CNV formation. In that context OCTA helps differentiating CNV from inflammatory tissue by demonstrating the hyperintense signal characteristic of CNV formation in the outer retina slab [3, 4].

2.1.1.1 Case presentation

A 58-year-old male presenting with bilateral diminution of vision of approximately 3 months duration. The patient reported more severe drop of vision in the left eye. He had history of previous similar attacks of visual disturbances in both eyes. His best-corrected visual acuity (BCVA) was 6/60 and 1/60 in the right and left eyes, respectively. Fundus examination of the right eye revealed multifocal serous retinal detachment in the posterior pole along with extensive sub-retinal exudate formation and optic nerve head (ONH) hyperemia. FFA revealed multiple leaking points at the level of the RPE with pooling of dye into the sub-retinal space and hyperfluorescence of the ONH due to leakage from dilated optic disc vessels. Fundus examination of the left eye showed similar findings in the posterior pole in addition to a sub-macular greenish-yellow lesion that demonstrated early hyperfluorescence with minimal leakage and late staining suggestive of predominantly scarred CNV.

2.1.1.1.1 SS-OCT and SS-OCTA features

The corresponding SS-OCT scan of the right eye showed marked thickening of the choroid with secondary undulations of the overlying RPE layer. The sub-retinal space showed multiple loculi of serous fluid and complete disruption of the

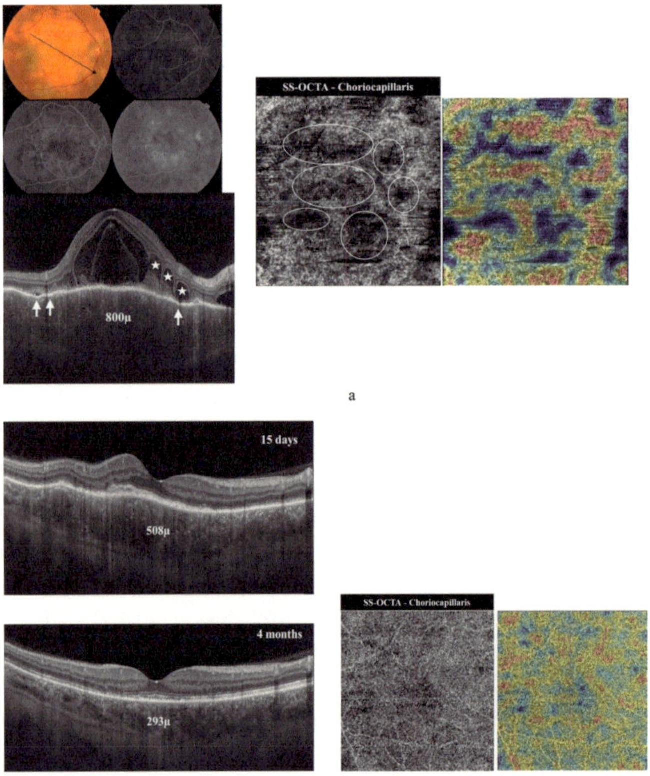

a

b

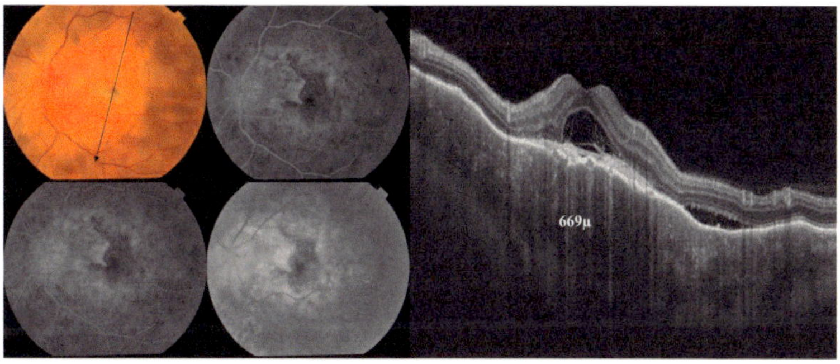

c

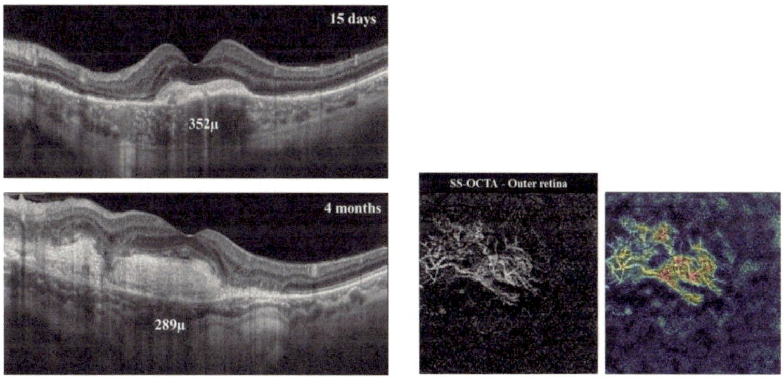

d

Figure 1.
(A) Top left: Color fundus photo and FFA of the right eye of a 58-year-old man presenting with acute attack of VKH. The posterior pole has a creamy yellowish appearance due to combination of multifocal neurosensory detachment and sub-retinal deposition of serous exudates. The ONH is hyperemic. FFA shows patchy choroidal filling persisting well into the venous phase, along with multiple pin-point leakage at the level of the RPE and diffuse hyperfluorescence due to pooling of dye into localized areas of neurosensory detachment. Bottom left: Radial scan SS-OCT shows marked increase in choroidal thickening (800 μm) and engorged choroidal vessels. Note the difficult delineation of the choroidal-scleral interface (CSI) due to optical hyporeflectivity secondary to engorged choroid. There are innumerable hyperreflective dots scattered within the choroid and possibly represent cellular inflammatory aggregates. The RPE shows multiple folds (white arrows). The neurosensory retina shows multiple hyporeflective loci separated by hyperreflective tissue septa (asterisks). Central macular thickness (CMT) is 970 μm. The hyporeflective loci are filled with hyperreflective amorphous material. There is complete disruption of the ellipsoid zone and outer retinal layers. Right: En-face SS-OCTA image of the choriocapillaris in a 6 × 6 mm field. Note the multiple discrete hypointense flow voids that are scattered within the choriocapillaris layer (white circles). The corresponding flow-density map shows blue color shades corresponding to the flow-void areas and denoting marked reduction of vessel density. (B) Radial scan SS-OCT images of the same patient at 15 days and 4 months after high-dose systemic steroid treatment. Note complete resolution of neurosensory detachment, and restoration of the ellipsoid zone. There is residual thickening of the RPE. Note improved delineation of the CSI and progressive disappearance of the previously seen hyperreflective dots in the choroid with resolution of choroidal inflammation. Bottom right: En-face SS-OCTA image of the choriocapillaris in a 6 × 6 mm field and the corresponding flow-density map at 4-month follow-up visit show significant recovery of the normal texture of the choriocapillaris denoting improvement of choriocapillaris perfusion. (C) Left: Color fundus photo and FFA of the left eye of the same patient. In addition to the features of acute stage of VKH, the macular area shows sub-retinal greenish-yellow lesion that demonstrates early minimal leakage on FFA and late staining suggestive of its predominant scar component. Right: Radial scan SS-OCT shows choroidal thickening (669 μm), blurred CSI, multiple neurosensory detachments with sub-retinal hyporeflective foci and hyperreflective amorphous deposits. Note the hyperreflective fusiform sub-foveal lesion. (D) Left: Radial scans SS-OCT during follow-up visits show resolution of the multifocal neurosensory detachment with persistence of the previously noted sub-retinal amorphous lesion. There is resolution of choroidal inflammation and improved visualization of the CSI. Bottom right: En-face SS-OCTA image and the corresponding flow-density map of the outer retina in a 6 × 6 mm field at 4-month follow-up visit show the hyperintense signal corresponding to high flow within neovascular complex. The abundant large mature vessels within the lesion denote a predominantly inactive CNV complex.

ellipsoid zone. SS-OCTA revealed loss of the normal hyperintense homogenous texture of the choriocapillaris and the development of moth-eaten like hypointense areas. SS-OCT examination of the left eye revealed large sub-foveal hyperreflective lesion with complete disorganization of the outer retinal layers and minimal overlying subretinal fluid, reminiscent of inactive type 2 CNV. SS-OCTA examination of the left eye confirmed inactive CNV formation. After receiving systemic steroid treatment the patient had complete resolution of the acute attack, with restoration of the normal retinal architecture and normal choroidal thickness in the right eye. BCVA in the right eye improved to 6/6 (**Figure 1(A)–(D)**).

2.1.1.2 Case presentation

A 16-year-old female presenting with bilateral diminution of vision of approximately 2 weeks duration. Her BCVA was 6/60 bilaterally. Fundus examination of both eyes revealed multifocal serous retinal detachment in the posterior pole along with yellowish sub-retinal exudate formation and ONH hyperemia. FFA revealed numerous leaking points at the level of the RPE with pooling of dye into the sub-retinal space and hyperfluorescence of the ONH due to leakage from dilated optic disc vessels. Five months after the patient received high-dose steroid therapy, the fundus of both eyes showed resolution of the previously noted neurosensory detachments and development of diffuse RPE and choroidal pigmentary disturbances. The macular area of the left eye showed a sub-retinal greenish lesion suggestive of CNV formation.

2.1.1.2.1 SS-OCT and SS-OCTA features

The corresponding SS-OCT scan of the right eye in the chronic stage showed residual neurosensory detachment with persistent thickening of the choroid. SS-OCT of the left eye showed sub-retinal hyperreflective amorphous lesion corresponding to the macular lesion seen in the color photo. SS-OCT was inconclusive in differentiating the sub-retinal inflammatory material from CNV due to similar optical reflectance properties of both lesions. On the other hand, SS-OCTA of the left eye decisively excluded CNV formation (**Figure 2(A)** and **(B)**).

2.1.2 Serpiginous choroiditis

Serpiginous choroiditis is an autoimmune disorder characterized by primary choriocapillaropathy in the form of progressive vascular occlusion of the choriocapillaris and possibly larger choroidal vessels with secondary ischemic damage of the RPE and neurosensory retina. The classic presentation of the acute form is single or multiple sub-retinal creamy-white lesions developing at the edge of the optic disc and wind in the posterior pole in a centripetal serpentine or helical pattern. Less typical variants of the disease that do not have a peripapillary component include macular serpiginous, and ampiginous choroiditis. The latter form has an initial benign clinical presentation reminiscent of acute posterior multifocal placoid pigment epitheliopathy, and later follows a relentless progressive course. Serpiginous choroiditis is bilateral with propensity to recurrence. Disease re-activation is characterized by development of newer lesions at the edges of old healed scars. Chronic stage is characterized by diffuse atrophy and disappearance of the choriocapillaris with subsequent secondary atrophy of the RPE and outer retina, scarring and RPE pigmentary disturbances [33, 34]. The resultant choroidal thinning and loss of choriocapillaris will cause alteration of the normal structural OCT features in the form of forward bowing of the choroid with loss of the normal bowl-shaped configuration and anterior displacement of the Sattler's vessel layer, hence development of diffuse irregular flow-voids and enhanced visualization of the medium and large-sized choroidal vessels on OCTA slab of the choriocapillaris [35–37]. The disease

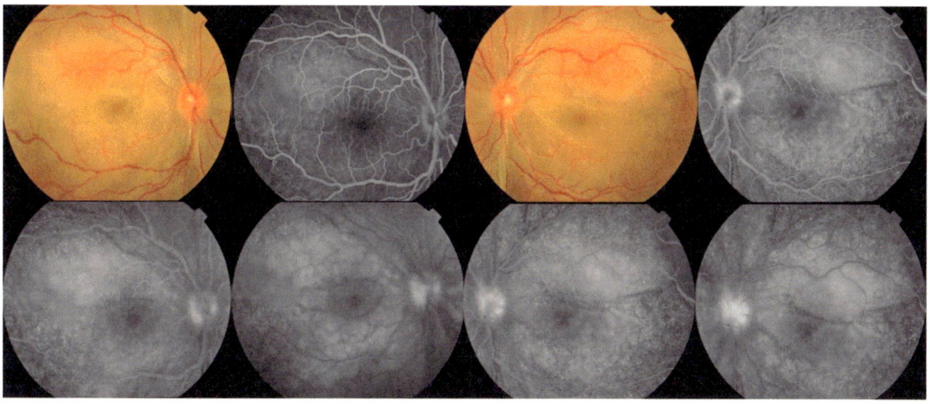

a

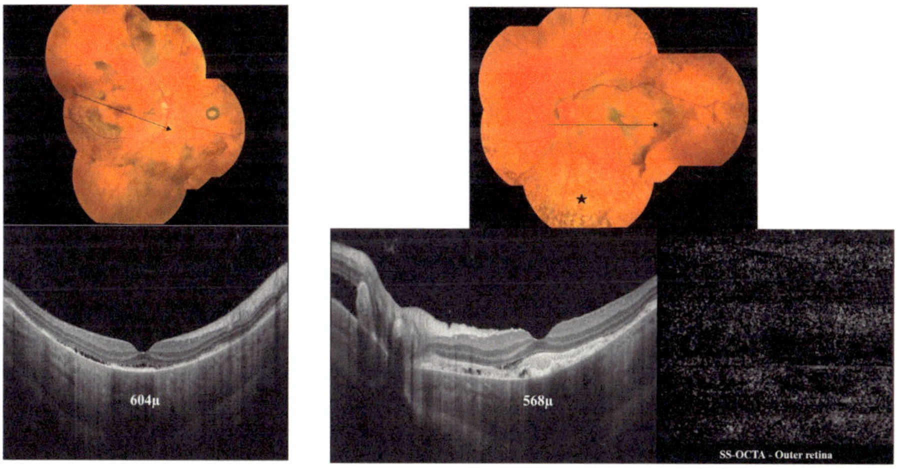

b

Figure 2.
(A) Color fundus photo and FFA of both eyes of a 16-year-old female with acute attack of VKH shows ONH hyperemia, and multiple neurosensory detachments with yellowish subretinal exudates. FFA demonstrates bilateral numerous leaking points at the level of the RPE. Note the classic starry-sky appearance that is characteristic of acute VKH. Later frames of FFA show pooling of dye into areas of multifocal neurosensory detachment, and ONH hyperfluorescence. (B) Top: Composite fundus photo of both eyes of the same patient 5 months later. The patient received high-dose systemic steroid treatment and developed chronic stage of VKH. Note the characteristic 'sunset glow' appearance of the fundus. Formation of Dalen-Fuchs nodules is more evident in the left eye (asterisk). Note the greenish sub-retinal lesion in the macular area in the left eye. Bottom left: High-definition line scan (12.0 mm) SS-OCT of the right eye shows irregular thickening of the RPE layer, sub-RPE and sub-retinal hyperreflective deposits, and residual neurosensory detachment. Note that the choroid is still grossly thickened. Bottom right: High-definition line scan (12.0 mm) SS-OCT of the left eye. Note the sub-foveal hyperreflective amorphous lesion corresponding to the macular lesion seen in the color photo. In this situation SS-OCT was inconclusive in excluding CNV formation. The corresponding en-face SS-OCTA image of the outer retina in a 6 × 6 mm field demonstrated normal hypointense appearance of an avascular outer retina, and decisively excluded CNV formation.

is notorious of aggressive course with propensity to involve the macular area and subsequent profound vision loss, which prompts briskly intervention with high-dose steroid therapy or other immunosuppressive agents for vision salvage [33].

2.1.2.1 Case presentation

A 28-year-old female patient who was a known case of bilateral serpiginous choroiditis. The patient presented with recent complaint of drop of vision approximately 1 month ago. Fundus examination in both eyes revealed large sharply circumscribed areas of sub-retinal fibrosis, with dense RPE clumps formation and variable degree of RPE pigmentary disturbances. Some of the lesions have coalesced together forming a continuum of sub-retinal scarring that involved almost the entire posterior pole. The distribution of the lesions was suggestive of previous episodes of classic form of serpiginous choroiditis. BCVA was counting fingers (CF) at 50 cm and 3/60 in the right and left eyes, respectively.

2.1.2.1.1 SS-OCT and SS-OCTA features

SS-OCT in both eyes showed marked thinning of the choroid with loss of the normal bowl-shaped configuration due to severe erosion of the choriocapillaris. The outer retina showed marked disorganization and atrophy. The RPE-Bruch's complex, external limiting membrane layer (ELM) and inner segment-outer segment photoreceptors junction (IS/OS) were replaced by amorphous hyper-reflective material. SS-OCTA showed irregular hypointense areas of flow-void amidst areas of preserved choriocapillaris denoting patchy loss of choriocapillaris (**Figure 3(A)** and **(B)**).

2.1.2.2 Case presentation

A 37-year-old female patient who was a known case of bilateral serpiginous choroiditis presenting for routine follow-up. BCVA was 6/60 and 6/36 in the right and left eyes, respectively. The posterior pole in both eyes showed large well-circumscribed areas of extensive chorioretinal atrophy involving the peripapillary area and extending into the macular region. The retinal layers and even underlying choroidal vasculature have virtually disappeared from wide areas of the lesion with unveiling of the underlying sclera.

2.1.2.2.1 SS-OCT and SS-OCTA features

SS-OCT in both eyes showed marked thinning of the fovea, and marked disorganization and atrophy of the outer retinal layers. The choroid showed diffuse loss of the choriocapillaris and of the larger choroidal vessels with subsequent loss of the normal bowl-shaped configuration. SS-OCTA showed diffuse loss of the choriocapillaris with unveiling of the larger choroidal vessels (**Figure 4(A)** and **(B)**).

2.1.3 Multifocal choroiditis (MFC) and punctate inner choroidopathy (PIC)

MFC and PIC are idiopathic chorioretinal inflammatory disorders that are grouped under the spectrum of white dot syndromes. The phenotypic features of both entities overlap in many aspects to the extent that they are considered variants of the same disorder rather than separate clinical entities. MFC/PIC have predilection for young myopic females. Their hallmark is the development of yellowish-white chorioretinal lesions scattered throughout the posterior pole and the periphery of the fundus. Histologically, these lesions are composed of aggregates of inflammatory cells beneath the RPE that cause multifocal conical elevation of the RPE cell layer in the form of inflammatory PED. These lesions eventually break-through the RPE into the sub-retinal space with subsequent release of the inflammatory infiltrates into the outer retina. Recurrent episodes of inflammation cause structural retinal damage. The chorioretinal pathologic cascade is associated with vitritis that is most marked in cases of MFC compared to PIC. As chronicity ensues these lesions develop into punched-out chorioretinal scars [38–41]. Secondary CNV formation is a frequent complication, mounting up to one-third of cases, though some studies report much higher incidence [42–44]. CNV superimposed

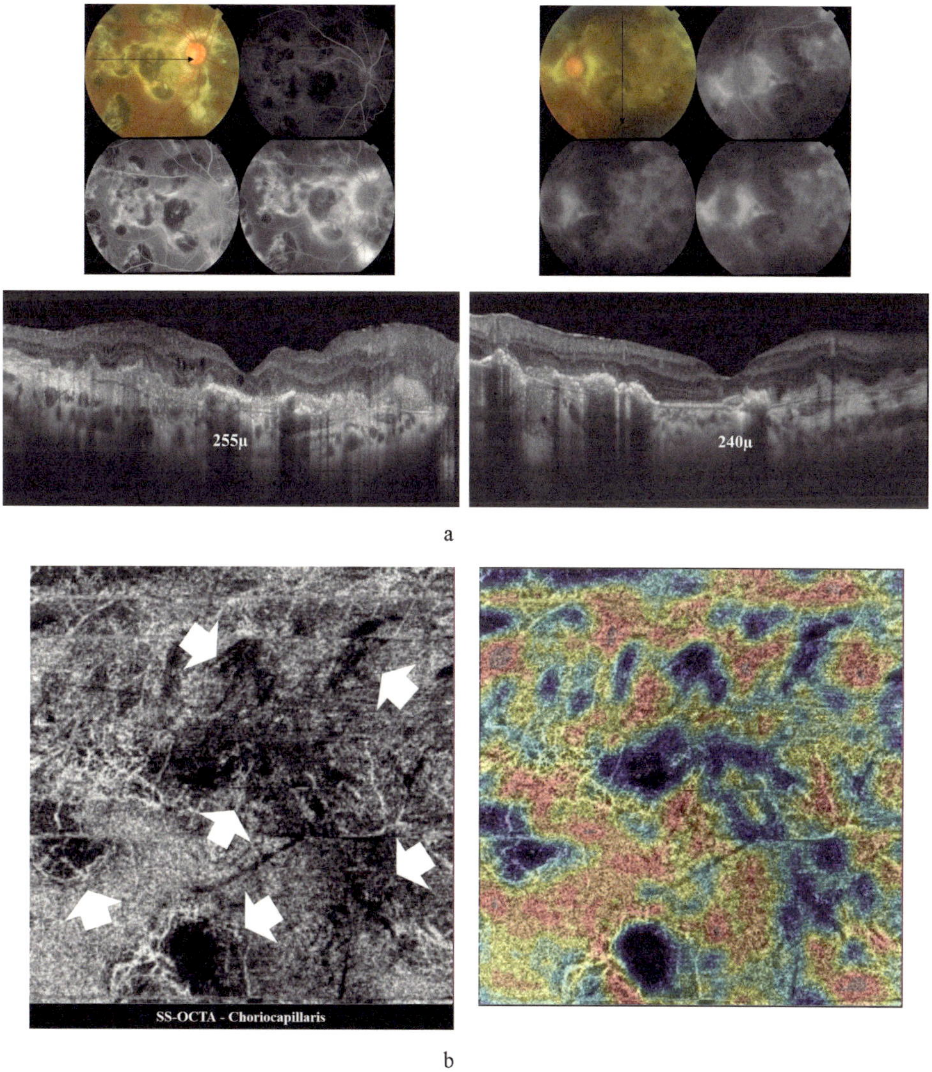

Figure 3.
(A) Top: Color fundus photo and FFA of both eyes of a 28-year-old female in chronic stage of serpiginous choroiditis. Note the diffuse plaques of sub-retinal fibrosis in the peripapillary area that radiate to involve almost the entire posterior pole. RPE pigment clumps formation is seen in the center of these lesions. On the corresponding FFA, these lesions show central blocked fluorescence surrounded by hyperfluorescent rim due to staining of the scar tissue. Bottom: Corresponding horizontal line scan (9.0 mm) SS-OCT (right), and vertical line scan (9.0 mm) SS-OCT (left) of both eyes show marked thinning of the choroid (255 and 240 μm in the right and left eyes, respectively). Note the irregular choroidal contour, marked thinning of the choriocapillaris and enhanced visualization of larger-sized choroidal vessels. The RPE-Bruch's complex, ellipsoid zone, ELM and IS/OS could not be identified and are replaced by amorphous hyper-reflective deposits. Note the foveal thinning and marked disorganization of the overlying neurosensory retina. (B) En-face SS-OCTA image and the corresponding flow density map of the choriocapillaris of the right eye in a 3 × 3 mm field. There are scattered sharply circumscribed areas of flow-voids due to loss of choriocapillaris (white arrows) with corresponding blue shades on the flow-density map. Note the enhanced visualization of the hyperintense signal of the larger choroidal vessels at the edges of the flow-voids and elsewhere due to combination of compensatory dilatation and anterior displacement of Sattler's vessel layer.

on MFC/PIC is usually a type 2 variant and is notoriously difficult to detect or to follow-up its response to anti-vascular endothelial growth factor (anti-VEGF) agents using conventional angiography techniques or structural OCT because it is characterized by minimal leakage on angiography and fluid accumulation on OCT, in addition to overlapping angiographic and OCT features with MFC/PIC-induced inflammation [10].

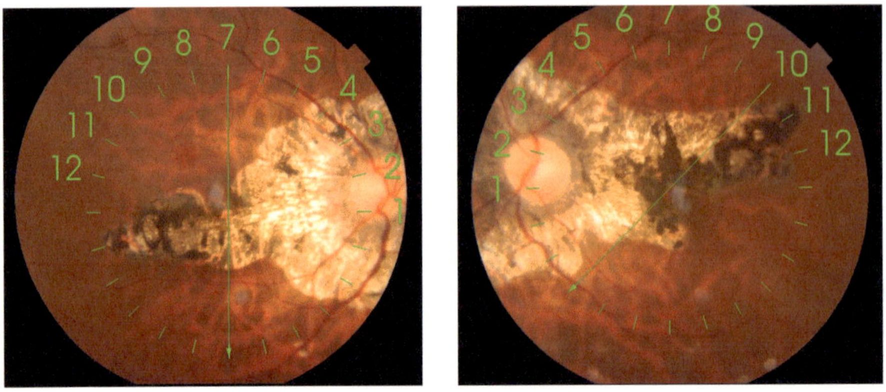

a

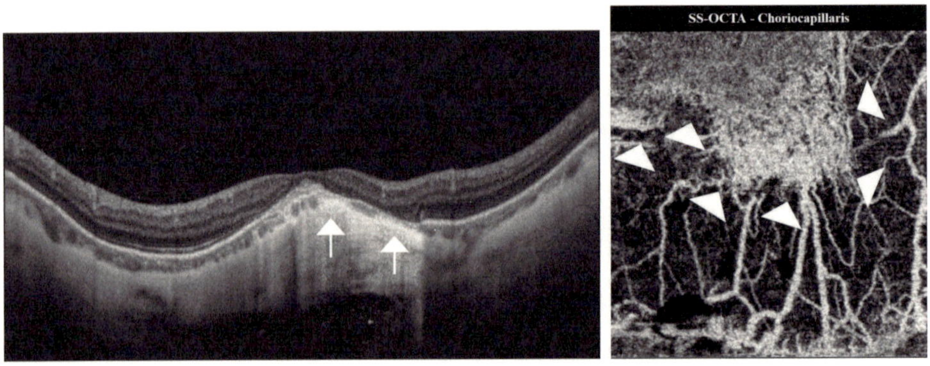

b

Figure 4.
(A) Color fundus photo of both eyes of a 37-year-old female with advanced posterior pole scarring secondary to serpiginous choroiditis. The retinal layers and underlying choroidal vasculature have virtually disappeared from the peripapillary and macular areas with secondary RPE pigment clumps formation. (B) Left: Radial scan SS-OCT of the right eye. Note almost complete disappearance of the choriocapillaris. The larger-sized choroidal vessel layer is thinned and has even disappeared in some areas (white arrows). In the sub-foveal area, a combination of severe atrophy of the neurosensory retina, RPE, choriocapillaris and marked anterior bowing of the choroid has resulted in enhanced optical reflectance of the choroid and underlying sclera. Right: Corresponding en-face SS-OCTA image at the level of the choriocapillaris in a 3 × 3 mm field. The choriocapillaris has been reduced to a small patch (white arrowheads) with near complete wiping of remaining parts and readily visualization of the larger choroidal vessels.

2.1.3.1 Case presentation

A 37-year-old female who is a known case of PIC presenting with drop of vision in the right eye of approximately 2-month duration. BCVA was 5/60 and 6/12 in the right and left eyes, respectively. Fundus examination of the right eye revealed features of myopic fundus with multiple discrete punched-out sub-retinal lesions scattered in the posterior pole and extending towards the equator. Most lesions were yellowish-white in color, whereas few lesions demonstrated variable degree of pigmentation. The foveal area showed a grayish sub-retinal lesion that exhibited typical features of classic CNV on FFA. SS-OCT confirmed the presence of type 2 CNV. SS-OCTA demonstrated hyperintense signal and characteristic features of active CNV. The patient received anti-VEGF injections for the right eye. At this stage her left fundus showed tessellated appearance with peripapillary atrophy due to myopia without signs of PIC. The patient returned 9 months later with complaints of metamorphopsia in the left eye. BCVA in the left eye has dropped to 6/18. Fundus examination revealed multiple scattered sub-retinal creamy white lesions. She was started on oral steroid therapy and the fundus lesions went onto remission though metamorphopsia persisted. Three months later she presented with worsening metamorphopsia and more drop of vision. BCVA in the left eye was 6/36. FFA, SS-OCT, and SS-OCTA revealed presence of CNV.

2.1.3.1.1 SS-OCT and SS-OCTA features

SS-OCT showed sub-RPE hyperreflective knob-like projections either confined to the sub-RPE space or breaking through into the sub-retinal space. SS-OCTA of the choriocapillaris revealed scattered foci of flow-voids corresponding to the location of the scarred punched-out lesions in the fundus. The foveal lesion suggestive of neovascular growth on color fundus photo and on FFA appeared as a sub-foveal amorphous hyperreflective material above the RPE suggestive of type 2 CNV with minimal overlying fluid. SS-OCTA at the level of the outer retina confirmed the hyperintense signal of flow within neovascular complex (**Figures 5(A)** and **(B)** and **6(A)** and **(B)**).

2.1.3.2 Case presentation

A 31-year-old female who is a known case of MFC presented with drop of vision in the left eye of approximately 3 weeks duration. BCVA was 6/6 and 3/60 in the right and left eyes, respectively. Fundus examination in the left eye revealed a sub-foveal yellowish-white lesion approximately 1 disc diameter (DD) in size. The posterior pole temporal to the lesion showed sub-retinal punched-out healed lesions of old episode of MFC. FFA demonstrated sub-foveal classic CNV formation. SS-OCT and SS-OCTA confirmed presence of neovascular growth. The patient started anti-VEGF injection that caused regression of the CNV. Her BCVA in the left eye after 3 ranibizumab injections and 7-month follow-up was 6/24.

2.1.3.2.1 SS-OCT and SS-OCTA features

SS-OCT examination revealed the presence of type 2 CNV with minimal overlying sub-retinal fluid. SS-OCTA revealed the hyperintense signal characteristic of flow within active neovascular network. On follow-up visits after the patient received anti-VEGF intravitreal injections, the morphology of the CNV on SS-OCT showed minimal variation. On the other hand, SS-OCTA was conclusive in documenting the regression of the CNV in response to anti-VEGF treatment (**Figure 7(A)** and **(B)**).

2.2 Infectious uveitides

2.2.1 Toxoplasmosis

Ocular toxoplasmosis is an infectious granulomatous posterior uveitis. The disease is considered the most common cause of posterior uveitis worldwide. Ocular involvement occurs as part of systemic toxoplasmosis. Infection is either congenital via transplacental transmission of the protozoan *Toxoplasma gondii* form an infected mother, or acquired due to ingestion of contaminated water or food or ingestion of undercooked meat containing toxoplasma cysts [45]. The clinical presentation is in the form of focal necrotizing retinochoroiditis in the posterior pole. The lesion can develop de novo or can present in the form of a satellite lesion, which is an acute focus of retinochoroiditis developing adjacent to an old chorioretinal scar. The lesion is associated with overlying vitritis which could be severe enough to obscure visualization of the fundus apart from the yellowish-white necrotizing focal lesion giving rise to the characteristic spotlight-in-the-fog appearance. As the acute episode subsides, a quiescent hyperpigmented scar

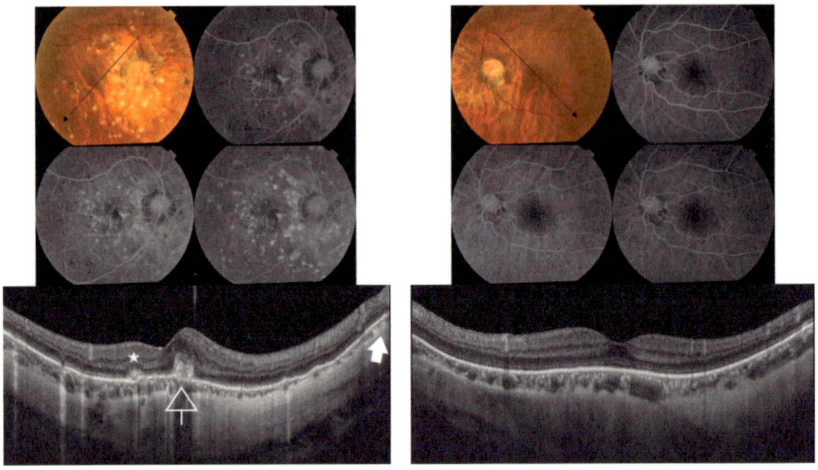

a

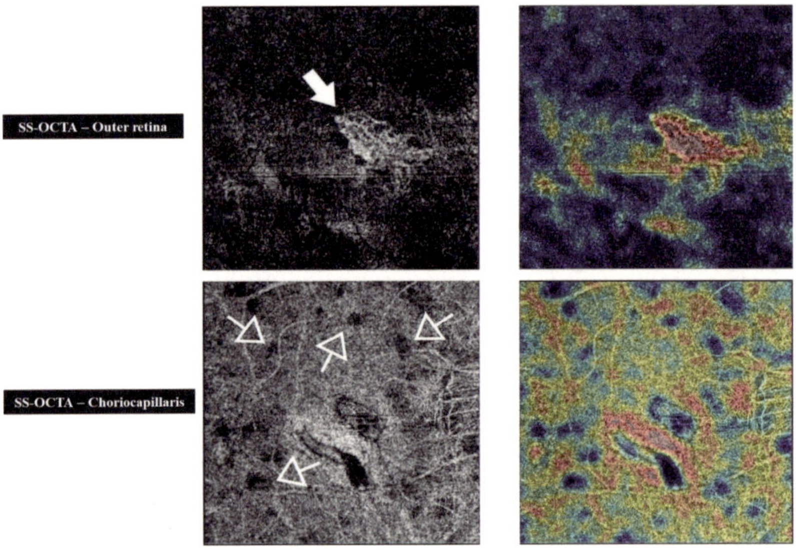

b

Figure 5.
(A) Top: Color fundus photo and FFA of the right and left eyes, respectively of a 37-year-old female with PIC. The right fundus shows multiple yellowish-white punched-out lesions scattered in the posterior pole and extending towards the equator. Some of these lesions show RPE clump deposition. The foveal area shows a sub-retinal grayish lesion. The fundus shows features of myopia as tessellated appearance and peripapillary chorioretinal atrophy. On FFA, the punched-out lesions seen in the color photo demonstrate early hyperfluorescence that gradually increases in intensity throughout successive frames due to combined pooling in PED and late staining. The lesions maintain sharply circumscribed boundaries without leakage of dye. Some of these lesions show blocked fluorescence due to masking by RPE clump formation. The foveal lesion shows early hyperfluorescence that gradually increases in intensity throughout successive frames due to minimal leakage. Color fundus photo and FFA of the left eye show myopic features. Bottom left: Radial scan SS-OCT of the right eye shows knob-like projections in the sub-RPE space (white arrow). One of these projections broke through into the sub-retinal space (asterisk). Note the sub-foveal hyperreflective amorphous lesion with minimal overlying fluid, suggestive of type 2 CNV formation (open arrow). Bottom right: Radial scan SS-OCT of the left eye showed choroidal thinning due to myopia. (B) Top: En-face SS-OCTA image in a 3 × 3 mm field at the level of the outer retina and the corresponding flow-density map show the hyperintense signal characteristic of flow within neovascular tissue (white arrow). The CNV shows dense arborization and anastomosis, which are characteristic of activity. Bottom: En-face SS-OCTA image in a 6 × 6 mm field at the level of the choriocapillaris and the corresponding flow-density map show the moth-eaten appearance of the choriocapillaris due to presence of scattered flow-voids (white open arrows) denoting foci of vascular atrophy and that correspond to the location of the punched-out lesions seen in the color photo.

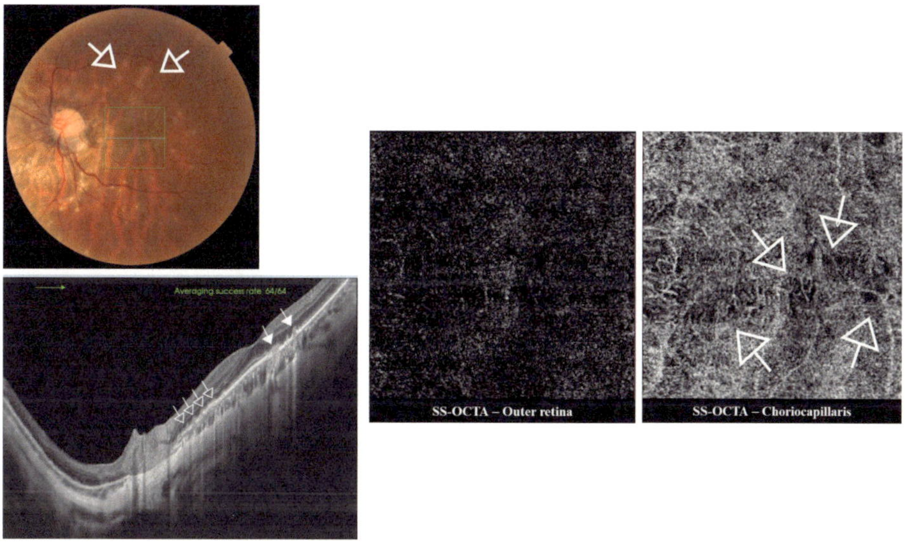

a

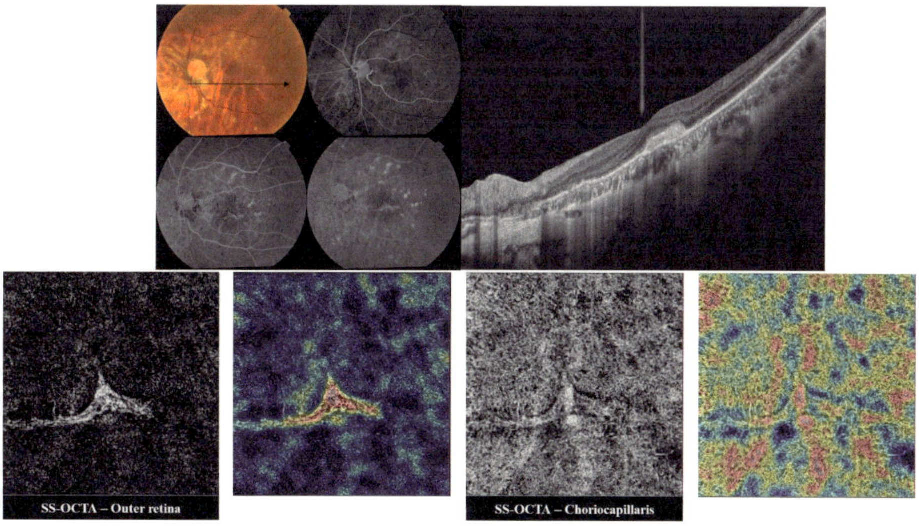

b

Figure 6.
(A) Top left: Color photo of the left fundus of the same patient in ***Figure 5****. Note the multiple creamy white lesions that developed in the posterior pole. Note the indistinct boundaries of some of these lesions (white open arrows), which indicate their recent onset compared to the atrophic punched-out appearance of the older lesions seen in the right fundus. Right: En-face SS-OCTA images in a 3 × 3 mm field of the outer retina and of the choriocapillaris. Note the normal appearance of the avascular outer retina, and the development of multiple foci of flow-voids in the choriocapillaris corresponding to the sub-retinal lesions seen in color photo. Bottom left: High-definition line scan (12.0 mm) SS-OCT of the left eye. Note the newly developed hyperreflective knob-like projections of the RPE cell layer (white open arrows). Some of these projections broke through the RPE into the sub-retinal space (white closed arrows). (B) Top left: Color fundus photo and FFA of the same patient 3 months later. Note the newly developed neovascular membrane in the foveal area. Top right: Radial scan SS-OCT shows newly developed sub-foveal hyperreflective amorphous lesion above the RPE, suggestive of type 2 CNV formation. Bottom left: En-face SS-OCTA image and the corresponding flow-density map of the outer retina in a 3 × 3 mm field show the hyperintense signal of the newly developed CNV. The dense arborization and anastomosis within the lesion are indicators of activity. Bottom right: En-face SS-OCTA image and the corresponding flow-density map of the choriocapillaris in a 3 × 3 mm field show multifocal hypointense signal due to flow-voids, which could result from multifocal atrophy of choriocapillaris due to older lesions or from signal masking in newer ones.*

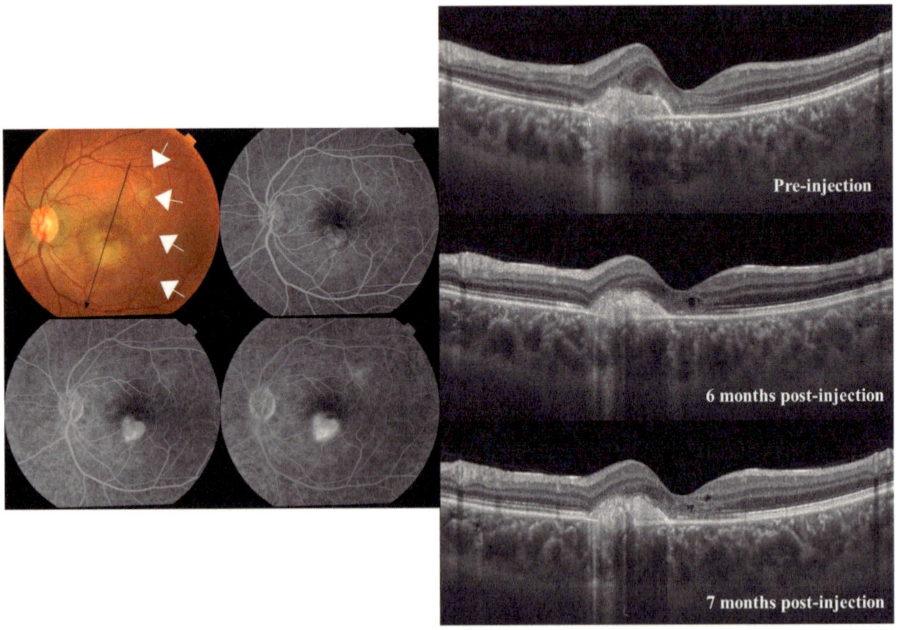

A

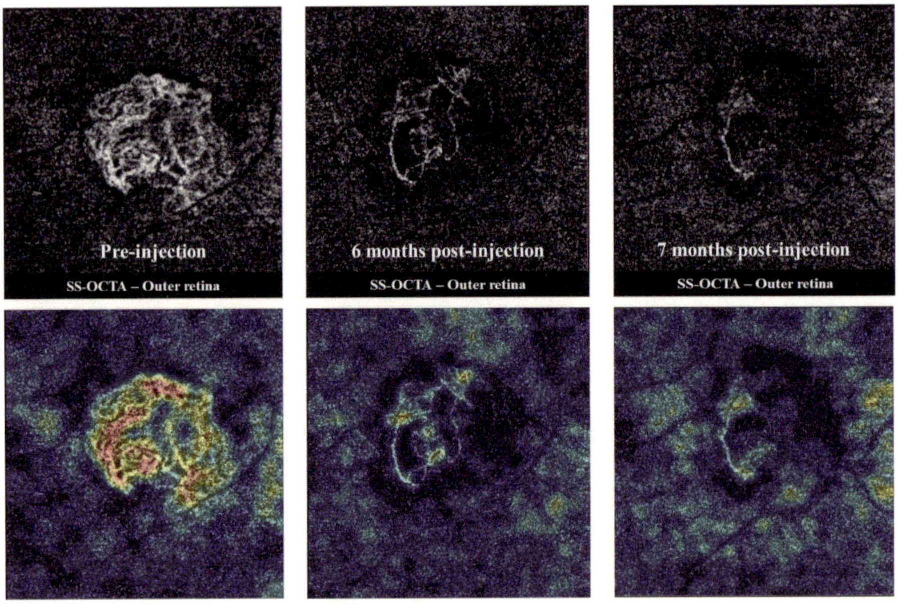

B

Figure 7.
(A) Left: Color fundus photo and FFA of the left eye of a 31-year-old female with MFC complicated by CNV formation. The fundus shows a sub-foveal yellowish-white lesion approximately 1 DD in size. Note the multiple whitish punched-out lesions located temporally and denote healed MFC lesions (white arrows). On FFA, the sub-foveal lesion demonstrates early well-circumscribed hyperfluorescence with late profuse leakage beyond the boundaries of the lesion. Right: Radial scan mode SS-OCT shows hyperreflective amorphous lesion lying entirely above the RPE with minimal overlying hyporeflective sub-retinal fluid. Note the minimal variation in the lesion morphology in follow-up SS-OCT scans, hence inconclusive information on CNV response to therapy. (B) En-face SS-OCTA images of the outer retina and the corresponding flow-density maps in a 3 × 3 mm field at initial presentation (left) and during follow-up visits after receiving anti-VEGF treatment (middle and right). At presentation, SS-OCTA of the outer retina demonstrated the hyperintense signal characteristic of flow within neovascular growth. Note the extensive anastomosis and dense arborization within the lesion, which indicate active CNV. Note the unequivocal SS-OCTA depiction of gradual regression of the CNV lesion during follow-up visits in response to anti-VEGF treatment.

develops which could lead to profound visual loss should it affect the macula or the papillomacular bundle [18]. On structural OCT, an active lesion features thickening and disorganization of the neurosensory retina, thickening of the choroid underlying the lesion and evidence of vitritis in the form of hyperreflective dots and thickening of the posterior hyaloid. As the lesion heals, the patient develops a chorioretinal scar with marked thinning and disorganization of the neurosensory retina and thinning of the underlying choroid. Choroidal neovascularization and vitreoretinal interface disturbances in the form of vitreoretinal tractional bands can develop [17, 18, 46].

2.2.1.1 Case presentation

A 13-year-old male presented to our clinic complaining of diminution of vision in his right eye of 3 days duration. Fundus examination revealed whitish retinal lesion inferonasal to the ONH with feathery indistinct edges and overlying vitritis. The ONH was inflamed with blurred edges. BCVA was 6/60 and 6/6 in the right and left eyes, respectively. Due to proximity of the lesion to the optic disc and the macula, we started the patient on oral sulfadiazine, pyrimethamine, and folinic acid. Oral steroids were started 24 h after initiation of antimicrobial regimen. At 2-month follow-up visit, the fundus showed resolution of previously noted vitritis and disc hyperemia, and regression of the retinal lesion, which appeared smaller in size and had well-defined boundaries. BCVA in the right eye improved to 6/6.

2.2.1.1.1 SS-OCT and SS-OCTA features

SS-OCT showed focal thickening with complete disorganization of the neurosensory retina, disruption of the ELM, IS/OS, and RPE cell layer with focal thickening of the choroid beneath the lesion. The overlying vitreous showed dense infiltration with hyperreflective foci indicating vitritis. SS-OCTA showed localized hypointense signal in the SCP, DCP, and choriocapillaris corresponding due to the masking by the focal lesion. During follow-up the previously noted hypointense signal regressed in size in proportion to regression of the lesion (**Figure 8(A)** and **(B)**).

2.2.1.2 Case presentation

A 26-year-old female presented to our clinic complaining of diminution of vision in her right eye of 1 week duration. Fundus examination revealed yellowish-white retinal lesion composed of a larger focus and smaller adjacent lesions overlying the papillomacular bundle. BCVA was 6/24 and 6/6 in the right and left eyes, respectively. As the lesion involved the papillomacular bundle, the patient was started on oral sulfadiazine, pyrimethamine, and folinic acid. Oral steroids were started 24 h after initiation of antimicrobial regimen.

2.2.1.2.1 SS-OCT and SS-OCTA features

SS-OCT showed focal thickening with complete disorganization of the neurosensory retina, disruption of the ELM, IS/OS, and RPE cell layer with focal thickening of the choroid beneath the lesion. The posterior hyaloid was thickened and partially attached to the focal retinal lesion. SS-OCTA showed localized hypointense signal in the SCP, DCP, and choriocapillaris corresponding to the masking effect of the focal lesion (**Figure 9(A)** and **(B)**).

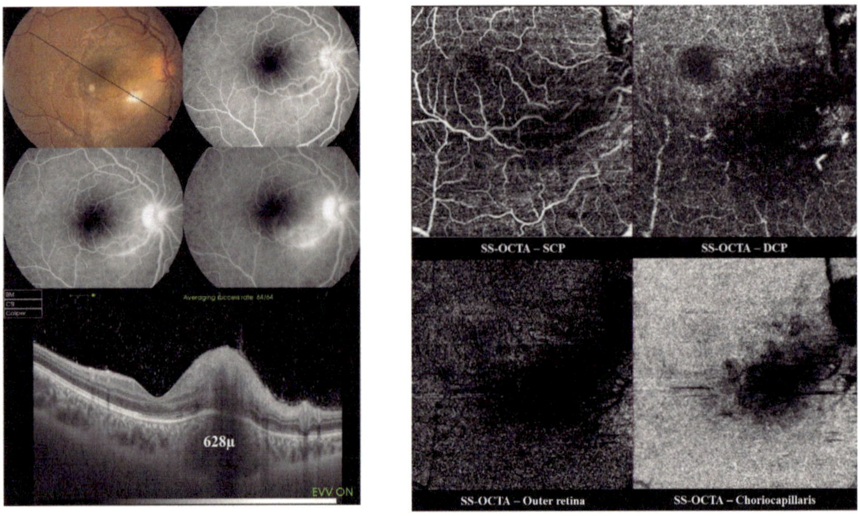

a

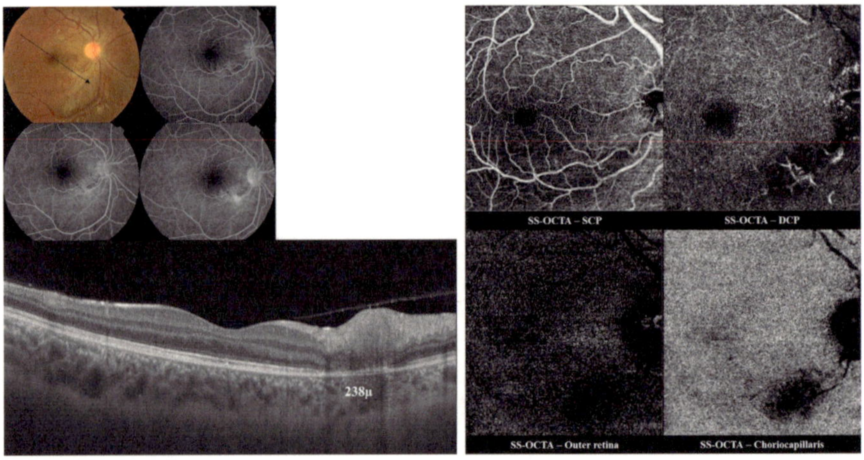

b

Figure 8.
(A) Top left: Color fundus photo and FFA of the right eye of a 13-year-old male with acute toxoplasma retinochoroiditis. The fundus shows a whitish retinal lesion inferotemporal to ONH with blurred edges and overlying vitritis. The ONH shows hyperemia and engorged peripapillary vessels. The corresponding FFA shows early localized blocked fluorescence corresponding in size and location to the lesion seen in color photo. Later frames show leakage from adjacent focal retinal vasculitis. The ONH demonstrates hyperfluorescence due to leakage form inflamed optic disc vessels. Bottom left: High-definition line scan (12.0 mm) SS-OCT shows focal thickening of the retina temporal to the optic disc with marked disorganization of the retinal layers and increased optical reflectance giving the affected part a blurred hyperreflective appearance known as the smudge effect, and causing optical shadowing of the underlying choroid. Note focal disruption of the ELM, and IS/OS layers in the area of the lesion. The choroid underlying the focal lesion is markedly thickened (628 μm), with focal blurring of the CSI. The overlying vitreous shows dense infiltration with hyperreflective foci, which represent inflammatory cell infiltrates. Right: En-face SS-OCTA images in a 6 × 6 mm field of the SCP, DCP, outer retina, and the choriocapillaris show hypointense signal caused by masking of the vascular layers and overshadowing of the outer retina by the focal lesion and overlying vitreous opacity. (B) Top left: Color fundus photo and FFA of the right eye at 2-month follow-up visit. Note resolution of vitritis, optic disc swelling, and a smaller size well-defined residual lesion. The corresponding FFA shows significantly improved retinal vasculitis and minimal leakage from the optic disc vessels. Bottom left: Radial scan SS-OCT shows complete resolution of choroidal inflammation (choroidal thickening measured 238 μm), with a well-defined CSI. The previously noted hyperreflective foci in the vitreous disappeared almost completely. There is significant improvement in the previously noted focal thickening of the retina, though with persistent disorganization of retinal layers and disruption of ELM and IS/OS layers. Top right: En-face SS-OCTA images of the SCP, DCP, outer retina, and the choriocapillaris in a 6 × 6 mm field show marked regression of the previously noted hypointense signal and improved visualization of the normal architecture of the vascular layers and of the outer retina.

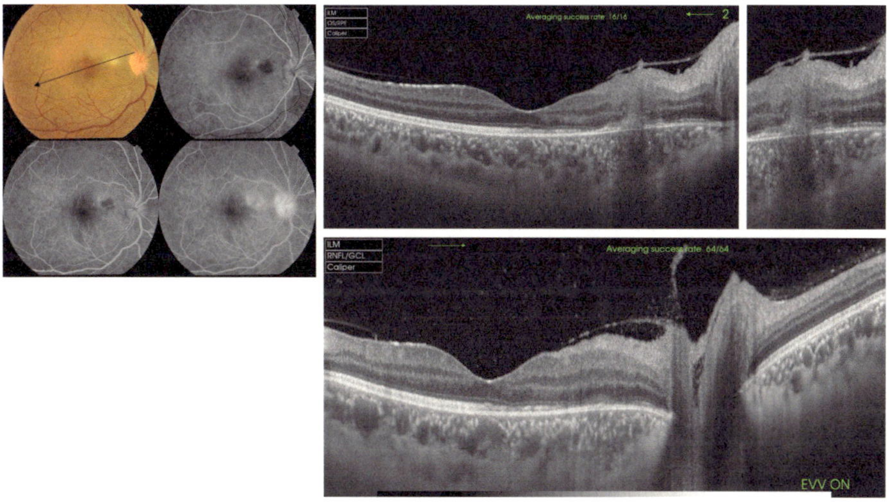

a

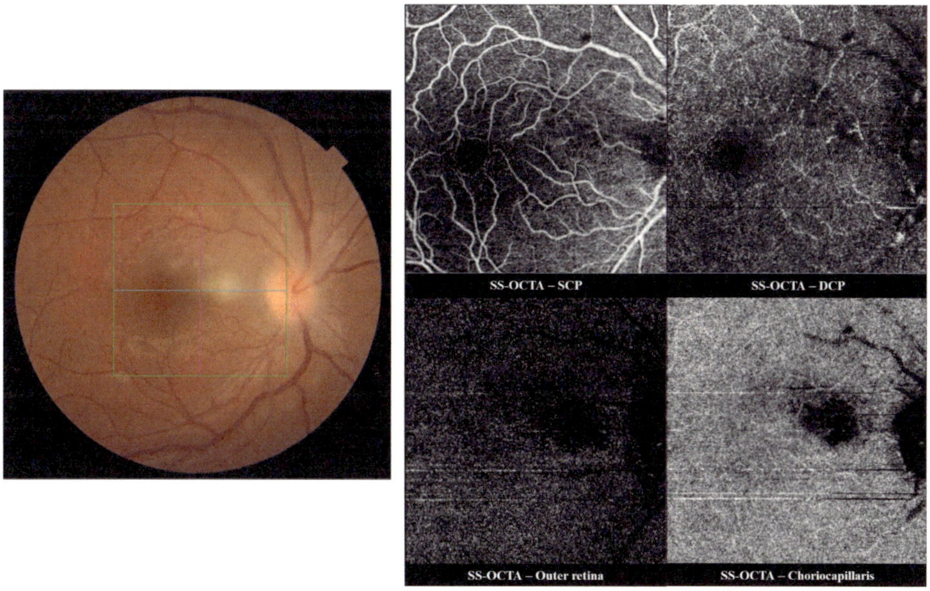

b

Figure 9.
(A) Top left: Color fundus photo and FFA of the right eye of a 26-year-old female with acute toxoplasma retinochoroiditis. Note the yellowish-white lesions overlying the papillomacular bundle that consist of a single larger focus and adjacent smaller ones. The partially blurred appearance of the optic disc and the papillomacular bundle is caused by vitritis overlying the lesion. FFA shows localized blocked fluorescence corresponding in size and location to the lesion seen in color photo. In later frames, leakage from adjacent focal retinal vasculitis causes hyperfluorescence. The ONH demonstrates hyperfluorescence due to leakage from inflamed disc vessels. Top middle: Radial scan SS-OCT shows focal thickening of the retina temporal to the optic disc with marked disorganization of the retinal layers and increased optical reflectance giving the affected part a blurred hyperreflective appearance known as the smudge effect, and causing optical shadowing of the underlying choroid. The ELM, IS/OS layers are disrupted. The choroid underlying the focal lesion is thickened. The overlying vitreous shows thickening of the posterior hyaloid which is partially attached to the focal retinal lesion. Top right: A zoom-in on the attachment between the focal retinal lesion and the posterior hyaloid. Bottom: High-definition line scan (12.0 mm) SS-OCT with the enhanced vitreous visualization (EVV) mode turned-on. Note the multiple hyperreflective dots scattered in the vitreous cavity and deposited along the posterior hyaloid face. (B) En-face SS-OCTA images of the SCP, DCP, outer retina and the choriocapillaris in a 6 × 6 mm field show hypointense signal caused by masking of the vascular layers and overshadowing of the outer retina by the focal lesion.

2.2.1.3 Case presentation

A female child, 8 years old presented to our office. Her mother reported noticing deviation of the right eye of her child and poor vision upon covering the left eye. BCVA was HM and 6/6 in the right and left eyes, respectively. Fundus examination of the right eye revealed a large saucer-shaped deeply excavated pigmented chorioretinal scar occupying the macular area.

2.2.1.3.1 SS-OCT and SS-OCTA features

SS-OCT showed marked thinning and disorganization of the retina, irregular elevation and thickening of the RPE and altered choroidal contour. SS-OCTA showed complete loss of the choriocapillaris at the site of the scar with unveiling of the large choroidal vessels underneath (**Figure 10**).

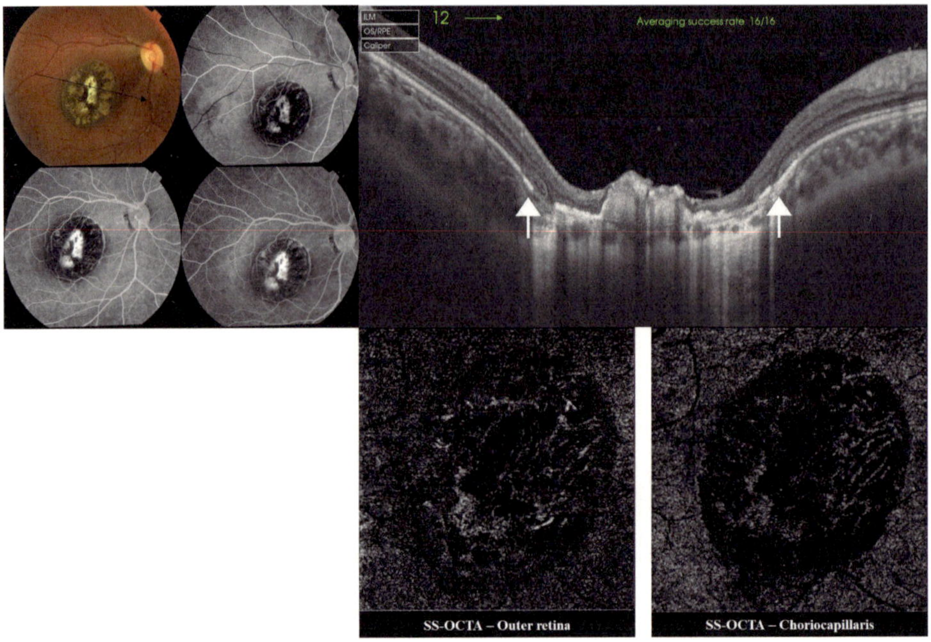

Figure 10.
Top left: Color fundus photo and FFA of the right eye of an 8-year-old female child with old toxoplasmosis scar. The macular area is almost entirely occupied by a large oval chorioretinal scar with sharply-circumscribed edges. The lesion shows variable grades of RPE pigmentary disturbances. The central part of the lesion shows complete chorioretinal atrophy exposing the underlying sclera. Note that the scar is sharply focused in comparison to the slightly defocused ONH and peripapillary area, which indicates the deeper plane of the scar due to excavation. On FFA, the lesion shows alternating areas of blocked fluorescence due to RPE pigment clumps formation and hyperfluorescence due to staining of scar tissue. Top right: Radial scan SS-OCT of the macular area. Note the abrupt transition from normal retinal layers at the edges of the lesion (white arrows) to marked thinning and disorganization of the neurosensory retina in the scar area. The central part of the lesion shows lumpy hyperreflective amorphous lesion representing the thickened distorted RPE layer. The underlying choroid is markedly thinned with increased optical reflectivity due to enhanced light penetration through the over-thinned layers. Bottom: En-face SS-OCTA images of the outer retina and choriocapillaris. The overthinning of the retina, and loss of choriocapillaris at the site of chorioretinal scar led to enhanced visualization of the Sattler's layer in the choriocapillaris and outer retina slabs.

3. Conclusion

The introduction of SS-OCT and SS-OCTA technology greatly propelled the management course of uveitis by unveiling previously unexplored areas of retinal and choroidal pathological morphology in uveitides, and by introducing new inflammatory biomarkers that helped monitoring the disease response to various therapeutic agents. The non-invasive nature of the new technology added to its versatility in particular clinical situations in which conventional angiography could be impractical or hazardous especially in lengthy follow-up protocols, pediatric patients, pregnant females, and patients with severely compromised renal function. However, this nascent technology should be considered an important complimentary tool to conventional angiographic tests without substituting them. Conventional FFA and ICG still maintain the lead role in diagnosis of uveitides by providing yet unmatched information on *leakage* which is by far the most important biomarker in monitoring the state of inner blood-retina-barrier in inflammatory entities as uveitides.

Author details

Magdy Moussa[1,2*] and Mahmoud Leila[3]

1 Ophthalmology, Ophthalmology Department, Faculty of Medicine, Tanta University, Tanta, Egypt

2 MEDIC Eye Center, Tanta, Egypt

3 Ophthalmology, Retina Department, Research Institute of Ophthalmology, Giza, Egypt

*Address all correspondence to: magdymoussa60@gmail.com

References

[1] Richard G, Soubrane G, Yannuzzi LA. The principles of fluorescein angiography. In: Fluorescein and ICG Angiography. Textbook and Atlas. 2nd ed. New York: Thieme; 1998. pp. 66-101

[2] Staurenghi G, Bottoni F, Giani A. Clinical applications of diagnostic indocyanine green angiography. In: Ryan SJ, editor. Retina. 6th ed. Philadelphia: Saunders; 2018. pp. 46-76

[3] Pichi F, Sarraf D, Morara M, Mazumdar S, Neri P, Gupta V. Pearls and pitfalls of optical coherence tomography angiography in the multimodal evaluation of uveitis. Journal of Ophthalmic Inflammation and Infection. 2017;**7**:20. DOI: 10.1186/s12348-017-0138-z

[4] Agarwal A, Invernizzi A, Singh RB, Foulsham W, Aggarwal K, Handa S, et al. An update on inflammatory choroidal neovascularization: Epidemiology, multimodal imaging, and management. Journal of Ophthalmic Inflammation and Infection. 2018;**8**:13. DOI: 10.1186/s12348-018-0155-6

[5] Bonnin S, Mané V, Couturier A, et al. New insight into the macular deep vascular plexus imaged by optical coherence tomography angiography. Retina. 2015;**35**:2347-2352

[6] Coscas F, Glacet-Bernard A, Miere A, et al. Optical coherence tomography angiography in retinal vein occlusion: Evaluation of superficial and deep capillary plexa. American Journal of Ophthalmology. 2016;**161**:160-171

[7] Spaide RF, Klancnik JM Jr, Cooney MJ. Retinal vascular layers imaged by fluorescein angiography and optical coherence tomography angiography. JAMA Ophthalmology. 2015;**133**(1):45-50

[8] De Carlo TE, Romano A, Waheed NK, et al. A review of optical coherence tomography angiography (OCTA). International Journal of Retina and Vitreous. 2015;**1**:5

[9] Wang Q, Chan S, Yang JY, et al. Vascular density in retina and choriocapillaris as measured by optical coherence tomography angiography. American Journal of Ophthalmology. 2016;**168**:95-109

[10] Levison AL, Baynes KM, Lowder CY, Kaiser PK, Srivastava SK. Choroidal neovascularisation on optical coherence tomography angiography in punctate inner choroidopathy and multifocal choroiditis. The British Journal of Ophthalmology. 2017;**101**(5):616-622

[11] Grulkowski I, Liu JJ, Potsaid B, Jayaraman V, Lu CD, Jiang J, et al. Retinal, anterior segment and full eye imaging using ultrahigh speed swept source OCT with vertical-cavity surface emitting lasers. Biomedical Optics Express. 2012;**3**(11):2733-2751

[12] Stanga PE, Tsamis E, Papayannis A, Stringa F, Cole T, Jalil A. Swept-source optical coherence tomography angiography ™ (Topcon Corp, Japan): Technology review. Developments in Ophthalmology. 2016;**56**:13-17

[13] Ikuno Y, Maruko I, Yasuno Y, Miura M, Sekiryu T, Nishida K, et al. Reproducibility of retinal and choroidal thickness measurements in enhanced depth imaging and high-penetration optical coherence tomography. Investigative Ophthalmology & Visual Science. 2011;**52**:5536-5540

[14] Fong AHC, Li KKW, Wong D. Choroidal evaluation using enhanced depth imaging spectral-domain optical coherence tomography in Vogt-Koyanagi-Harada disease. Retina. 2011;**31**:502-509

[15] Maruko I, Iida T, Sugano Y, Oyamada H, Sekiryu T, Fujiwara T, et al. Subfoveal choroidal thickness after treatment of Vogt-Koyanagi-Harada disease. Retina. 2011;**31**:510-517

[16] Nakayama M, Keino H, Okada AA, Watanabe T, Taki W, Inoue M, et al. Enhanced depth imaging optical coherence tomography of the choroid in Vogt-Koyanagi-Harada disease. Retina. 2012;**32**:2061-2069

[17] Chen KC, Jung JJ, Engelbert M. Single acquisition of the vitreous, retina and choroid with swept-source optical coherence tomography in acute toxoplasmosis. Retinal Cases & Brief Reports. 2016;**10**:217-220

[18] Goldenberg D, Goldstein M, Loewenstein A, Habot-Wilner Z. Vitreal, retinal and choroidal findings in active and scarred toxoplasmosis lesions: A prospective study by spectral-domain optical coherence tomography. Graefe's Archive for Clinical and Experimental Ophthalmology. 2013;**251**:2037-2045

[19] Gao SS, Liu G, Huang D, Jia Y. Optimization of the split-spectrum amplitude-decorrelation angiography algorithm on a spectral optical coherence tomography system. Optics Letters. 2015;**40**(10):2305-2308

[20] Kuehlewein L, Tepelus TC, An L, Durbin MK, Srinivas S, Sadda SR. Noninvasive visualization and analysis of the human parafoveal capillary network using swept source OCT optical microangiography. Investigative Ophthalmology & Visual Science. 2015;**56**(6):3984-3988

[21] Savastano MC, Lumbroso B, Rispoli M. In vivo characterization of retinal vascularization morphology using optical coherence tomography angiography. Retina. 2015;**35**(11):2196-2203

[22] Spaide RF. Volume-rendered angiographic and structural optical coherence tomography. Retina. 2015;**35**:2181-2187

[23] Astroz P, Miere A, Mrejen S, Sekfali R, Souied EH, Jung C, et al. Optical coherence tomography angiography to distinguish choroidal neovascularization form macular inflammatory lesions in multifocal choroiditis. Retina. 2018;**38**:299-309

[24] Nakao S, Kaizu Y, Oshima Y, Sakamoto T, Ishibashi T, Sonoda KH. Optical coherence tomography angiography for detecting choroidal neovascularization secondary to punctate inner choroidopathy. Ophthalmic Surgery, Lasers and Imaging Retina. 2016;**47**(12):1157-1161

[25] Kotsolis AI, Killian FA, Ladas ID, Yannuzzi LA. Fluorescein angiography and optical coherence tomography concordance for choroidal neovascularization in multifocal choroiditis. The British Journal of Ophthalmology. 2010;**94**:1506-1508

[26] Vance SK, Khan S, Klancnik JM, Freund KB. Characteristics of spectral-domain optical coherence tomography findings of multifocal choroiditis. Retina. 2011;**31**:717-723

[27] Nussenblatt RB. Vogt-Koyanagi-Harada syndrome. In: Nussenblatt RB, Whitcup SM, editors. Uveitis. Fundamentals and Clinical Practice. 4th ed. Vol. 2010. USA: Mosby. pp. 303-318

[28] Goto H, Rao PK, Rao NA. Vogt-Koyanagi-Harada disease. In: Ryan SJ, editor. Retina. 6th ed. Philadelphia: Saunders; 2018. pp. 1505-1515

[29] Baltmr A, Lightman S, Tomkins-Netzer O. Vogt-Koyanagi-Harada syndrome—Current perspectives. Clinical Ophthalmology. 2016;**10**:2345-2361

[30] Rao NA. Pathology of Vogt-Koyanagi-Harada disease. International Ophthalmology. 2007;**27**:81-85

[31] Aggarwal K, Agarwal A, Deokar A, Mahajan S, Singh R, Bansal R, et al. Distinguishing features of acute Vogt-Koyanagi-Harada disease and acute central serous chorioretinopathy on optical coherence tomography angiography and en face optical coherence tomography imaging. Journal of Ophthalmic inflammation and infection. 2017;**7**(3). DOI: 10.1186/s12348-016-0122-z

[32] Aggarwal K, Agarwal A, Mahajan S, Invernizzi A, Mandadi SKR, Singh R, et al. The role of optical coherence tomography angiography in the diagnosis and management of acute Vogt-Koyanagi-Harada disease. Ocular Immunology and Inflammation. 2018;**26**(1):142-153

[33] Nussenblatt RB. Serpiginous choroidopathy. In: Nussenblatt RB, Whitcup SM, editors. Uveitis. Fundamentals and Clinical Practice. 4th ed. Vol. 2010. USA: Mosby. pp. 373-382

[34] Pakzad-Vaezi K, Khaksari K, Chu Z, Van Gelder RN, Wang RK, Pepple KL. Swept-source OCT angiography of serpiginous choroiditis. Ophthalmology Retina. 2018;**2**:712-719

[35] Ahn SJ, Park SH, Lee BR. Multimodal imaging including optical coherence tomography angiography in serpiginous choroiditis. Ocular Immunology and Inflammation. 2017;**25**(2):287-291

[36] El Ameen A, Herbort CP Jr. Serpiginous choroiditis imaged by optical coherence tomography angiography. Retinal Cases & Brief Reports. 2018;**12**(4):279-285

[37] Mandadi SKR, Agarwal A, Aggarwal K, Moharana B, Singh R, Sharma A, et al. Novel findings on optical coherence tomography angiography in patients with tubercular serpiginous-like choroiditis. Retina. 2017;**37**:1647-1659

[38] Amer R, Louis N. Punctate inner choroidopathy. Survey of Ophthalmology. 2011;**56**:36-53

[39] Essex RW, Wong J, Jampol LM, Dowler J, Bird AC. Idiopathic multifocal choroiditis: A comment on present and past nomenclature. Retina. 2013;**33**:1-4

[40] Spaide RF, Goldberg N, Freund KB. Redefining multifocal choroiditis and panuveitis and punctate inner choroidopathy through multimodal imaging. Retina. 2013;**33**:1315-1324

[41] Zahid S, Chen KC, Jung JJ, Balaratnasingam C, Ghadiali Q, Sorenson J, et al. Optical coherence tomography angiography of chorioretinal lesions due to idiopathic multifocal choroiditis. Retina. 2017;**37**:1451-1463

[42] Nussenblatt RB. White-dot syndromes. In: Nussenblatt RB, Whitcup SM, editors. Uveitis. Fundamentals and Clinical Practice. 4th ed. Vol. 2010. USA: Mosby. pp. 383-400

[43] Patel KH, Birnbaum AD, Tessler HH, Goldstein DA. Presentation and outcome of patients with punctate inner choroidopathy at a tertiary referral center. Retina. 2011;**31**:1387-1391

[44] Campos J, Campos A, Mendes S, Neves A, Beselga D, Sousa JPC. Punctate inner choroidopathy: A systematic review. Medical Hypothesis, Discovery & Innovation Ophthalmology. 2014; **3**(3):76-82

[45] Belfort R Jr, Silveira C, Muccioli C. Ocular toxoplasmosis. In: Ryan SJ, editor.

Retina. 6th ed. Philadelphia: Saunders; 2018. pp. 1681-1684

[46] Oréfice JL, Costa RA, Campos W, Calucci D, Scott IU, Oréfice F. Third-generation optical coherence tomography findings in punctate retinal toxoplasmosis. American Journal of Ophthalmology. 2006;**142**

Chapter 7

OCT Findings in Myopic Traction Maculopathy

Ramesh Venkatesh, Bharathi Bavaharan and Naresh Kumar Yadav

Abstract

The prevalence of myopia is constantly on a rise. Patients with high myopia and pathological myopia can lose vision due to a number of degenerative changes occurring at the macula. With recent advances in imaging techniques such as spectral domain optical coherence tomography (OCT) and swept-source OCT, our understanding of macular pathology in myopia has improved significantly. New conditions such as myopic traction maculopathy have been identified and defined. Treatment approaches are now being planned on the basis of the pathoanatomy of myopic traction maculopathy on OCT. In this chapter, we discuss the role of OCT imaging in myopic traction maculopathy.

Keywords: myopia, traction maculopathy, posterior staphyloma

1. Introduction

Myopic traction maculopathy was first described by Panozza and associates in 2004 as a group of pathological features seen in eyes with high myopia generated by traction [1]. In recent times, MTM is also termed as myopic foveoschisis. One of the important reasons for reduced vision in these myopic eyes is traction-related retinal disorders. Eyes with myopic traction maculopathy demonstrate features of vitreomacular traction, retinal thickening, macular retinal schisis-like thickening, lamellar macular hole (MH), and foveal retinal detachment (FRD)[2]. Many of these retinal pathologies are not detectable on clinical examination and are only found on advanced imaging with optical coherence tomography. Because of the clinical subtlety of some of these disorders, decreased visual acuity may be attributed to other causes, whereas macular traction may remain undiagnosed [3–8]. The natural course of myopic macular traction disorders is not clear. Some studies have shown progression to more serious complications like full-thickness MH and FRD while a few studies have shown spontaneous resolution of foveal detachment and macular retinoschisis after development of spontaneous posterior vitreous detachment (PVD) [6, 9–13]. Optical coherence tomography (OCT) is a useful, non-invasive and indispensable tool in the diagnosis, pathogenesis, staging, prognosis, treatment and follow-up of MTM. In this article, we describe the role of OCT imaging in MTM.

IntechOpen

2. Pathogenesis

Before the advent of OCT, the anatomic features of MTM were not described and the pathogenesis was poorly understood. Both TD-OCT and SD-OCT studies have provided an invaluable contribution to the characterization and understanding of the underlying pathologic mechanism involved in MTM. There are four major traction mechanisms identified in MTM: (1) Peri foveal vitreomacular traction (2) Cortical vitreous remnants after (PVD) development (3) Epiretinal membrane formation (4) Intrinsic non-compliance of the internal limiting membrane (ILM) and inner retina to conform to the shape of the posterior staphyloma [14, 15]. The first three mechanisms constitute the extrinsic forces (outside the retina) responsible for MTM while the stiff ILM and inner retinal layers constitute the intrinsic force (within the retina) responsible for MTM formation. The ILM itself can cause traction in eyes with posterior staphyloma.

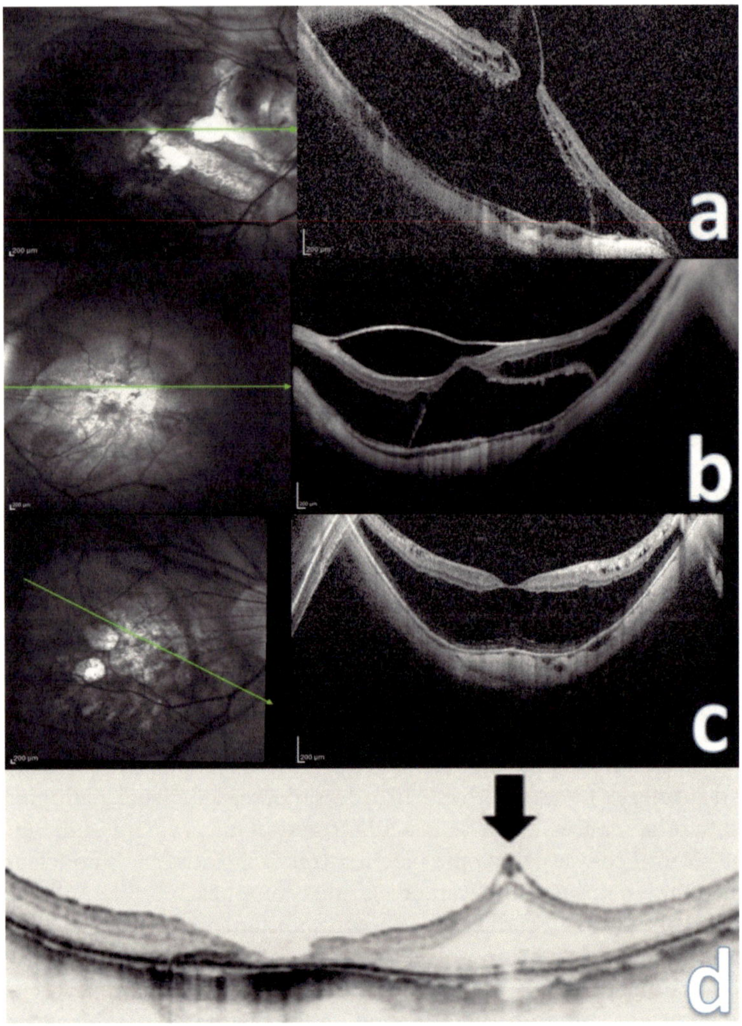

Figure 1.
Mechanisms causing MTM. (a) MTM caused by vitreomacular traction with presence of foveal retinal detachment (FRD). (b) Epiretinal membrane causing schisis-like retinal thickening with associated FRD. (c) MTM with no apparent preretinal membranes. (d) Tenting of the inner retina at the retinal arteriole (black arrow) with complete resolution of the retinal thickening following vitrectomy in MTM.

It appears that in eyes without identifiable preretinal tractional elements, ILM peeling resolves the retinal thickening. There are two possible explanations: One is that the ILM is highly elastic and tough, rendering it taut like a drum. In eyes with posterior staphyloma, the ILM is like the surface of a drum and is relatively resistant to permanent deformation and stretching. The second, more probable, explanation is that microscopic cellular and collagen proliferation develops on the ILM surface after PVD causing the ILM to be less distensible and making it more rigid. This prevents the ILM to conform to the contour of the posterior staphyloma and causes a schisis-like retinal thickening [16]. Understanding the pathogenetic mechanism responsible for MTM formation helps in deciding the surgical approach in these eyes (**Figure 1**).

3. Diagnosis

Myopic tractional maculopathy is virtually seen in eyes with posterior staphyloma. In a study using SD-OCT, Henaine-Berra et al. [17] identified MTM in 17 of 116 eyes of pathological myopia, thus reporting a prevalence of approximately 15%. Some of these retinal changes are difficult to appreciate in eyes with high myopia due to the presence of the pathological degenerative changes at the posterior pole. Decreased visual acuity in these eyes is usually attributed to causes other than macular traction. OCT is often used in identifying the different retinal pathologies like vitreomacular traction, retinal thickening, macular retinoschisis, lamellar MH, and FRD. Progression of the myopic tractional detachment to develop a full-thickness MH and macular retinal detachment can also be identified with use of OCT.

4. Staging and classification

On the basis of OCT, Shimada et al. [4] have classified MTM into five stages from S0 to S4. This staging is based on the location of retinoschisis and its extent of macular involvement (**Table 1**).

Shimada et al. [4] further defined the progression as an increase of the extent or height of retinoschisis (more than 100 μm) or the development of an inner lamellar MH, FRD, or full-thickness MH. During a mean follow-up of 36.2 months, they reported progression in 11.6% (24/207) eyes, which included 0.9% who progressed to full-thickness MH and 3.4% who progressed to FRD. The eyes with extensive macular retinoschisis (S4) showed progression significantly more (42.9%) than eyes having less extensive macular retinoschisis areas (6.7%). Six (21.4%) of 28 eyes with S4 MTM progressed to foveal detachment (**Figures 2** and **3**).

Stage	Location and involvement
0	No retinoschisis
1	Extrafoveal
2	Foveal
3	Both foveal and extrafoveal but not the entire macula
4	Entire macula

Table 1.
Staging of myopic tractional maculopathy depending on the extent of involvement.

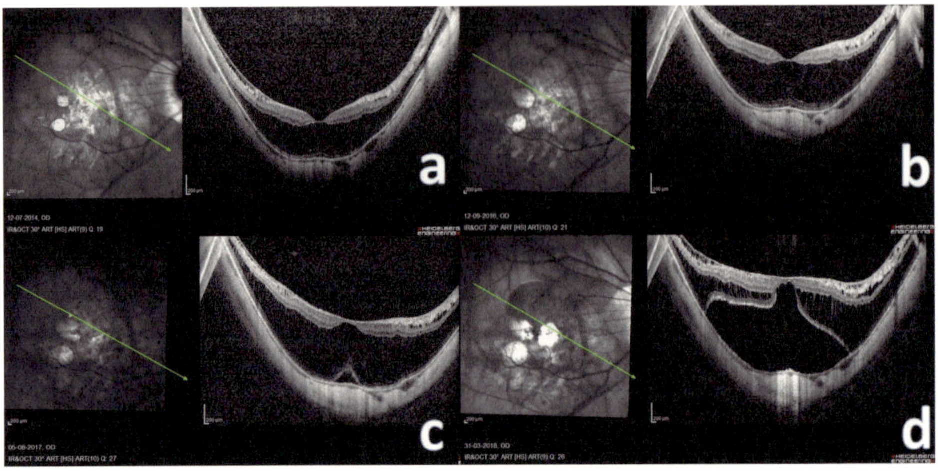

Figure 2.
(a–d) Progression of MTM leading to FRD over a period of 5 years.

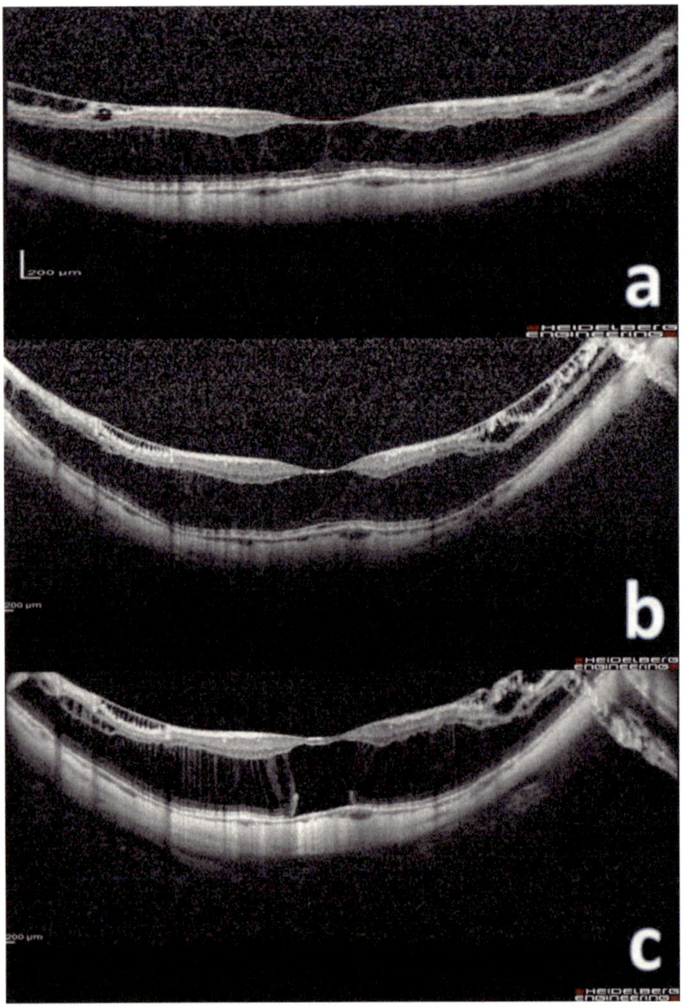

Figure 3.
(a–c) Progression of MTM in the fellow eye of a patient who had undergone vitrectomy for MTM with foveal detachment in the other eye.

5. Treatment

The goal of treatment in MTM is to relieve the tractional forces responsible for the formation of MTM [18]. This can be achieved primarily with the help of internal procedure with vitrectomy and external procedure with macular buckle. Pharmacologic vitreolysis can be considered a useful treatment option if vitreomacular traction from the perifoveal PVD or traction associated with a remnant cortical vitreous layer after PVD is responsible for the MTM formation.

The indications of surgery in MTM are:

1. Recent onset reduction in visual acuity secondary to development of full-thickness MH or FRD.

2. Progression in the extent of the schisis-like thickening documented by OCT.

3. Vision <20/50.

Most surgeons while dealing with myopic traction maculopathy have two approaches:

1. Minimalist approach—This involves identifying and resolving only the major traction mechanism visible on OCT. In this approach, only vitrectomy with PVD induction is carried out. ILM peeling is not done in these cases. This avoids complications of ILM peeling in select eyes, but it is unlikely to be successful in each and every case.

2. Comprehensive approach—In this approach, all the preretinal tractional elements are removed along with ILM peeling in every case. This approach has the highest single-operation success rate and ensures complete removal of all cellular and vitreous components that might cause current or future traction [14].

Taniuchi et al. [19] evaluated the effect of vitrectomy with and without ILM peeling in 71 eyes of 64 patients with myopic traction maculopathy. They studied the effects on visual acuity and post-operative complications. The results indicated that vitrectomy with ILM peeling can lead to improvement in vision in patients with macular retinoschisis or foveal detachment. Recurrences of tractional macular detachment were also more frequent in eyes without ILM peeling.

5.1 Surgical techniques

Basically, vitrectomy with removal of the posterior cortical vitreous is what is minimally required in relieving the tractional forces responsible for MTM formation. The role of additional procedures like peeling of internal limiting membrane and use of gas tamponade in MTM is debatable. In eyes with MTM secondary to vitreomacular traction from the perifoveal PVD and traction associated with a remnant cortical vitreous layer after PVD, vitrectomy alone with removal of posterior cortical vitreous is sufficient in relieving the traction and achieves a normal retinal anatomy. In eyes with MTM secondary to epiretinal membrane formation, additional removal of epiretinal membrane is required. MTM caused by intrinsic stiffening of the ILM requires peeling of ILM with or without the placement of macular buckle [20, 21]. Few studies have shown that sparing a small island of ILM over the fovea in eyes with MTM can prevent the development of post-operative MHs which are usually difficult to fix [22, 23] (**Table 2**).

MTM	Surgery procedure
(1) Due to vitreomacular traction from the perifoveal PVD	Vitrectomy with posterior cortical vitreous removal
(2) Due to traction associated with a remnant cortical vitreous layer after PVD	Vitrectomy with posterior cortical vitreous removal
(3) Due to epiretinal membrane formation	Vitrectomy with posterior cortical vitreous removal with ERM removal
(4) Due to intrinsic stiffening of the ILM	(a) Vitrectomy with posterior cortical vitreous removal with ILM peeling (b) Macular buckle alone (c) combined vitrectomy and macular buckle
(5) With associated full-thickness MH or FRD	(a) Vitrectomy with posterior cortical vitreous removal with ILM peeling with gas tamponade (b) Macular buckle alone (c) Combined vitrectomy and macular buckle

Abbreviations: MTM—myopic traction maculopathy; PVD—posterior vitreous detachment; ERM—epiretinal membrane; ILM—Internal limiting membrane; MH—Macular hole; FRD—Foveal retinal detachment.

Table 2.
Surgical decision-making in myopic traction maculopathy based on pathoanatomy seen on optical coherence tomography.

Common difficulties encountered during vitrectomy in these high myopic eyes are: (1) inability of the smaller gauge instruments to reach the retinal tissue at the macula due to longer axial length; (2) In eyes with posterior staphyloma, the vitreous is strongly adherent to the edge of the staphyloma resulting in retinal breaks during PVD induction; (3) Staining of ILM with various dyes is usually inadequate and patchy making ILM peeling difficult in these scenarios; (4) Glaucoma is associated with high myopia resulting in an already compromised optic nerve head which can get worsened following vitrectomy; (5) Scleral thinning associated with high myopia

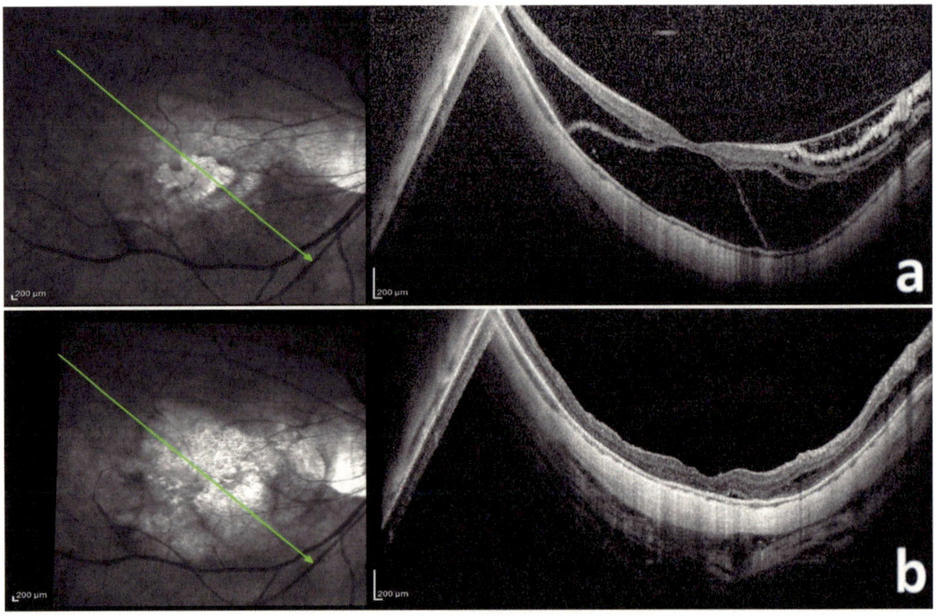

Figure 4.
(a–b) Pre and post-operative images of a patient with myopic foveoschisis with FRD. At 6 months post-op, there is complete resolution of the retinal thickening and subretinal fluid.

can lead to catastrophic complications like expulsive hemorrhage. Thus, macular buckle has emerged as a useful and effective treatment option in the management of MTM. However, due to the longer learning curve of this technique and unpredictable outcomes following this procedure, vitrectomy still remains the most preferred treatment modality amongst most vitreoretinal surgeons in the management of MTM.

6. Monitoring

Following surgery for MTM, resolution of retinal thickening and/or foveal detachment is monitored using OCT. Complete resolution of retinal thickness or subretinal fluid is achieved in 6–9 months after surgery [24] (**Figure 4**). Patients with high myopia and unilateral MTM require regular OCT monitoring of the fellow eye to assess progression to myopic pre-MTM [25].

7. Conclusion

One of the important causes for disturbed vision secondary to high myopia is MTM. It may be difficult to appreciate MTM on clinical examination with biomicroscopy. With the advent of OCT, the diagnosis of MTM and a posterior staphyloma can be made easily. Newer generation OCT imaging modalities have helped in the understanding the mechanism of myopic foveoschisis formation and help in deciding the treatment plan by the retinal surgeon. Early detection and referral to a retinal specialist for evaluation and treatment when appropriate may prevent further vision loss secondary to MH formation and/or retinal detachment.

Author details

Ramesh Venkatesh*, Bharathi Bavaharan and Naresh Kumar Yadav
Narayana Nethralaya, Bengaluru, India

*Address all correspondence to: vramesh80@yahoo.com

References

[1] Panozzo G, Mercanti A. Optical coherence tomography findings in myopic traction maculopathy. Archives of Ophthalmology. 2004;**122**(10):1455-1460

[2] Kanski JJ. Clinical Ophthalmology: A Systematic Approach. 6th ed. Oxford: Butterworth-Heinemann Elsevier Ltd.; 2007. p. 931

[3] Smiddy WE, Kim SS, Lujan BJ, et al. Myopic traction maculopathy: Spectral domain optical coherence tomographic imaging and a hypothesized mechanism. Ophthalmic Surgery, Lasers and Imaging. 2009;**40**:169-173

[4] Shimada N, Ohno-Matsui K, Baba T, et al. Natural course of macular retinoschisis in highly myopic eyes without MH or retinal detachment. American Journal of Ophthalmology. 2006;**142**:497-500

[5] Takano M, Kishi S. Foveal retinoschisis and retinal detachment in severely myopic eyes with posterior staphyloma. American Journal of Ophthalmology. 1999;**128**:472-476

[6] Benhamou N, Massin P, Haouchine B, et al. Macular retinoschisis in highly myopic eyes. American Journal of Ophthalmology. 2002;**133**:794-800

[7] Ikuno Y, Tano Y. Early MHs with retinoschisis in highly myopic eyes. American Journal of Ophthalmology. 2003;**136**:741-744

[8] Baba T, Ohno-Matsui K, Futagami S, et al. Prevalence and characteristics of FRD without MH in high myopia. American Journal of Ophthalmology. 2003;**135**:338-342

[9] Shimada N, Ohno-Matsui K, Yshida T, et al. Progression from macular retinoschisis to retinal detachment in highly myopic eyes is associated with outer lamellar hole formation. The British Journal of Ophthalmology. 2008;**92**(6):762-764

[10] Sun CB, Liu Z, Xue AQ, Yao K. Natural evolution from macular retinoschisis to full-thickness MH in highly myopic eyes. Eye (London, England). 2010;**24**(12):1787-1791

[11] Gaucher D, Haouchine B, Tadayoni R, et al. Long-term follow-up of high myopic foveoschisis: Natural course and surgical outcome. American Journal of Ophthalmology. 2007;**143**(3):455-462

[12] Ripandelli G, Rossi T, Scarinci F, et al. Macular vitreoretinal interface abnormalities in highly myopic eyes with posterior staphyloma: 5-year follow-up. Retina. 2012;**32**(8):1531-1538

[13] Polito A, Lanzetta P, Del Borrello M, Bandello F. Spontaneous resolution of a shallow detachment of the macula in a highly myopic eye. American Journal of Ophthalmology. 2003;**135**(4):546-547

[14] Johnson MW. Myopic traction maculopathy: Pathogenic mechanisms and surgical treatment. Retina. 2012;**32**(Suppl 2):S205-S210

[15] VanderBeek BL, Johnson MW. The diversity of traction mechanisms in myopic traction maculopathy. American Journal of Ophthalmology. 2012;**153**(1):93-102

[16] Yokota R, Hirakata A, Hayashi N, Hirota K, Rii T, Itoh Y, et al. Ultrastructural analyses of internal limiting membrane excised from highly myopic eyes with myopic traction maculopathy. Japanese Journal of Ophthalmology. 2018;**62**(1):84-91

[17] Henaine-Berra A, Zand-Hadas IM, Fromow-Guerra J, García-Aguirre G. Prevalence of macular anatomic abnormalities

in high myopia. Ophthalmic Surgery, Lasers and Imaging Retina. 2013;**44**(2):140-144

[18] Hattori K, Kataoka K, Takeuchi J, Ito Y, Terasaki H. Predictive factors of surgical outcomes in vitrectomy for myopic traction maculopathy. Retina. 2018;**38**(Suppl 1):S23-S30

[19] Taniuchi S, Hirakata A, Itoh Y, Hirota K, Inoue M. Vitrectomy with or without internal limiting membrane peeling for each stage of myopic traction maculopathy. Retina. 2013;**33**(10):2018-2025

[20] Alkabes M, Mateo C. Macular buckle technique in myopic traction maculopathy: A 16-year review of the literature and a comparison with vitreous surgery. Graefe's Archive for Clinical and Experimental Ophthalmology. 2018;**256**(5):863-877

[21] Susvar P, Sood G. Current concepts of macular buckle in myopic traction maculopathy. Indian Journal of Ophthalmology. 2018;**66**(12): 1772-1784

[22] Ho TC, Chen MS, Huang JS, et al. Foveola nonpeeling technique in internal limiting membrane peeling of myopic foveoschisis surgery. Retina. 2012;**32**:631-634

[23] Shimada N, Sugamoto Y, Ogawa M, Takase H, Ohno-Matsui K. Fovea-sparing internal limiting membrane peeling for myopic traction maculopathy. American Journal of Ophthalmology. 2012;**154**(4):693-701

[24] Kumar A, Ravani R, Mehta A, Simakurthy S, Dhull C. Outcomes of microscope-integrated intraoperative optical coherence tomography-guided center-sparing internal limiting membrane peeling for myopic traction maculopathy: A novel technique. International Ophthalmology. 2018;**38**(4):1689-1696

[25] Xia HJ, Wang WJ, Chen F, Wu Y, Cai ZY, Chen W, et al. Long-term follow-up of the fellow eye in patients undergoing surgery on one eye for treating myopic traction maculopathy. Journal of Ophthalmology. 2016;**2016**:2989086

Section 3

OCT in Glaucoma

Chapter 8

Role of Optical Coherence Tomography in the Evaluation and Management of Glaucoma

Baswati Sahoo and Julie Pegu

Abstract

Glaucoma is the leading cause of irreversible, yet preventable, blindness throughout the world. Since it is a disease which can be treated but not cured, it is crucial for the treating ophthalmologist to catch the disease as early as possible. The diagnosis of glaucoma is currently based on the appearance of the optic disc and standard achromatic perimetry. However, to detect glaucoma in its early stages, there are various diagnostic modalities of which optical coherence tomography serves as a novel tool. Optical coherence tomography has emerged over the years with the ability to detect changes in the optic nerve head, retinal nerve fiber layer, and currently the ganglion cell layer much earlier than the defects manifest functionally. Thus, optical coherence tomography acts as an important diagnostic aid to diagnose and monitor the progression of this sight threatening disease called glaucoma.

Keywords: optical coherence tomography, pre perimetric glaucoma, ganglion cell complex, retinal nerve fiber layer, spectral domain optical coherence tomography, time domain optical coherence tomography

1. Introduction

From the early days until the turn of the twentieth century, glaucoma was defined as "pressure within the eye higher than the statistical normal of the population." It was thought that this rise in pressure caused damage to the optic nerve that was irreversible. It is not until the end of twentieth century, when newer concepts such as the ocular hypertension and the normal tension glaucoma emerged, which led people to challenge this definition [1]. Glaucoma then was redefined by the American Academy of Ophthalmology as an optic neuropathy with characteristic structural damage to optic nerve, associated with progressive retinal ganglion cell death, loss of nerve fibers, and visual field loss. However, the intraocular pressure was considered as the strongest risk factor and possibly the only modifiable one [2].

2. Why optic nerve?

Optic nerve evaluation is the cornerstone of management of glaucoma. It remains the most crucial step in the early diagnosis of glaucoma and monitoring progressive nerve damage. Stereoscopic changes in the optic nerve head and retinal nerve fiber layer, which are seen clinically, are actually the manifestations of loss

IntechOpen

of the ganglion cell layer which cannot be seen using slit lamp biomicroscopy. Moreover, since the structural abnormalities precede the functional changes, it is imperative to have an objective, quantitative, and reproducible imaging technique which is capable of early diagnosis and helps monitoring of the disease.

There are various imaging modalities being used by glaucoma experts today. Confocal scanning laser ophthalmoscopy (HRT; Heidelberg Retina Tomography; Heidelberg Engineering, Heidelberg, Germany), scanning laser polarimetry (GDX; Carl Zeiss Meditec, Dublin, California, USA), and optical coherence tomography (OCT; Carl Zeiss Meditec and others) are among the popular ones. However, subjective optic disc evaluation with stereo optic disc photography still remains the mainstay of every clinical practice.

3. Concept of preperimetric glaucoma

Glaucomatous optic neuropathy is characterized by structural changes in the optic disc in the form of thinning of neuroretinal rim, pallor, and progressive cupping of the optic disc. Since it is a disease which can be treated but not cured, it is crucial for the treating ophthalmologist to catch the disease in its early stages. In glaucoma, structural injury has been documented to precede functional injury in most eyes [3]. One of the reasons observed by many researchers was that it took almost a loss of 40% of the ganglion cells to pick up a defect on the standard automated perimetry. Recently, a change in the diagnostic criteria of glaucoma has been promoted so that glaucoma diagnosis may be made before the old prerequisites functional criteria of standard automatic perimetry visual field (SAP-VF) loss are apparent, namely the "preperimetric glaucoma" (PPG).

To be diagnosed as a case of PPG, a patient needs to have a structural injury to the optic nerve head (ONH) sufficient enough to be classified under glaucomatous optic neuropathy (GON) and ought to be clinically proven. The introduction of newer imaging devices such as confocal scanning laser ophthalmoscopy, scanning laser polarimetry, and optical coherence tomography for measuring structural changes in the optic nerve head and retinal nerve fiber layer seems promising for early detection of glaucoma. Although an effort has been made to diagnose glaucoma in its early stages, there is no evidence that a single measurement is superior to the others and a combination of tests may be needed for detecting early damage in glaucoma.

4. Diagnostic aids in preperimetric glaucoma

Standard automated perimetry is the gold standard in the diagnosis of glaucoma as it gives us an assessment of the functional loss occurring in glaucoma. Optic disc photography gives a structural assessment of the optic nerve and surrounding nerve fiber layer but can be challenging due to inter-individual variability. Serial 3D imaging on the other hand may seem to be a better way of the subjective diagnosis of glaucomatous optic neuropathy during its early stages [4, 5]. Capturing early loss of retinal nerve fibers both clinically and by means of red-free photos may not be easy and sometimes could be indecisive, particularly in diffuse than in localized retinal nerve fibers loss [6].

5. Optical coherence tomography (OCT)

Optical coherence tomography (OCT) is a non-invasive diagnostic technique that renders an *in vivo* cross-sectional view of the retina, retinal nerve fiber layer, and the

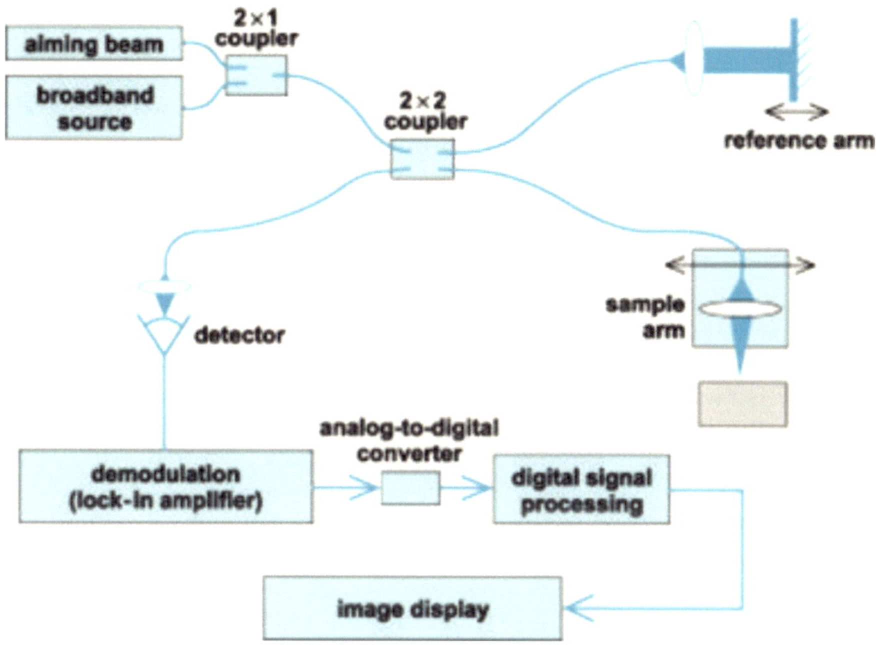

Figure 1.
Principle of optical coherence tomography.

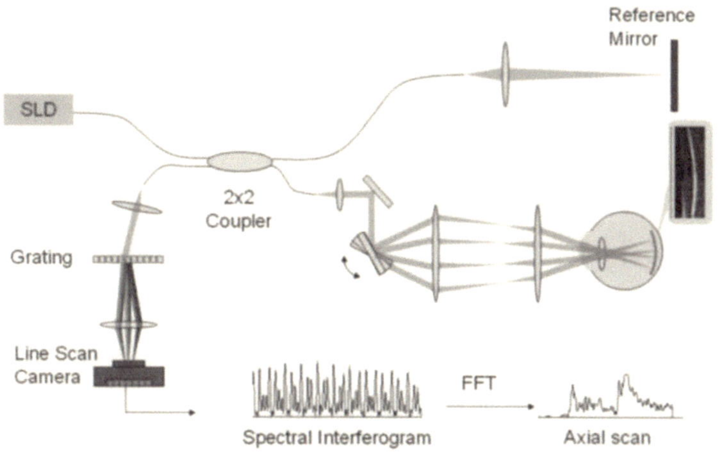

Figure 2.
Principle of Fourier domain optical coherence tomography.

optic nerve head. OCT utilizes a concept known as low coherence interferometry. A broadband width light from a superluminescent diode is projected onto the retina. This is divided into a reference and a sample beam, and further the echo time delays of light reflected from the retina as well as reference mirror at known distances is compared. The light waves that are backscattered from the retina, interfere with the reference beam, and this interference pattern is measured by a photodetector (**Figure 1**). This is the basic principle on which the Sratus OCT works.

Spectral domain OCT (SD-OCT) also works on similar principles, however, with a much higher data acquisition speed as compared to TD-OCT. This is achieved by the Michelson type interferometer with a stationary reference mirror. Instead of the interference signal being captured by a point detector, after the two returning beams recombine and form the interference pattern at the beam splitter, the interference pattern is split by a grating into its frequency components, all of these components are simultaneously detected by a charge-coupled device (CCD) (**Figure 2**). SD-OCT is also known as Fourier domain OCT (FD-OCT) because the distances are encoded in the Fourier transform of the frequencies of light reflected.

6. Spectrum of OCT in the diagnosis of glaucoma

The OCT can scan the optic nerve head (ONH), peripapillary retinal nerve fiber (RNFL), and the macular area (GCC—ganglion cell complex). An addition to the spectrum of posterior evaluation is the anterior segment OCT (AS-OCT) which utilizes a higher wavelength light to capture images of the anterior chamber angle.

7. Types of OCT

7.1 Stratus or time domain OCT

From its inception, OCT images were acquired in a time domain fashion. Time domain systems acquire approximately 400 A-scans per second using 6 radial slices oriented 30° apart. Time-domain OCT (TD-OCT) systems featured scan rates of 400 A-scans per second with an axial resolution of 8–10 μm in tissue [7]. Since the slices are 30° apart, there always is a possibility to miss pathology between the slices.

7.2 Fourier domain OCT (FD-OCT) or spectral domain OCT (SD-OCT)

SD-OCT, on the other hand, achieves scan rates of 20,000–52,000 A-scans per second and a resolution of 5–7 μm in tissue [8, 9]. This increased scan rate and number diminishes the likelihood of motion artifact, enhances the resolution, and decreases the chance of missing lesions.

7.3 Anterior segment OCT (AS-OCT)

Anterior segment OCT utilizes higher wavelength light (1310 nm) as compared to 830 nm of traditional posterior segment OCT. This higher wavelength light results in greater absorption and less penetration allowing clear images of the parts of the anterior segment (cornea, anterior chamber, iris, and angle). Currently, there are two commercially produced dedicated anterior segment devices, the slit lamp-OCT (SL-OCT: Heidelberg Engineering) and the Visante (Carl Zeiss Meditec, Inc.).

8. Clinical interpretation of OCT in glaucoma diagnosis

8.1 Stratus OCT (Carl Zeiss)

The Stratus OCT utilizes various protocols for analysis of the optic nerve head and the retinal nerve fiber layer.

8.1.1 Optic nerve head analysis

The "Fast Optic disc " pattern is used to analyze the optic nerve head. It consists of six evenly placed radial lines centered on the optic nerve head. Each of the six

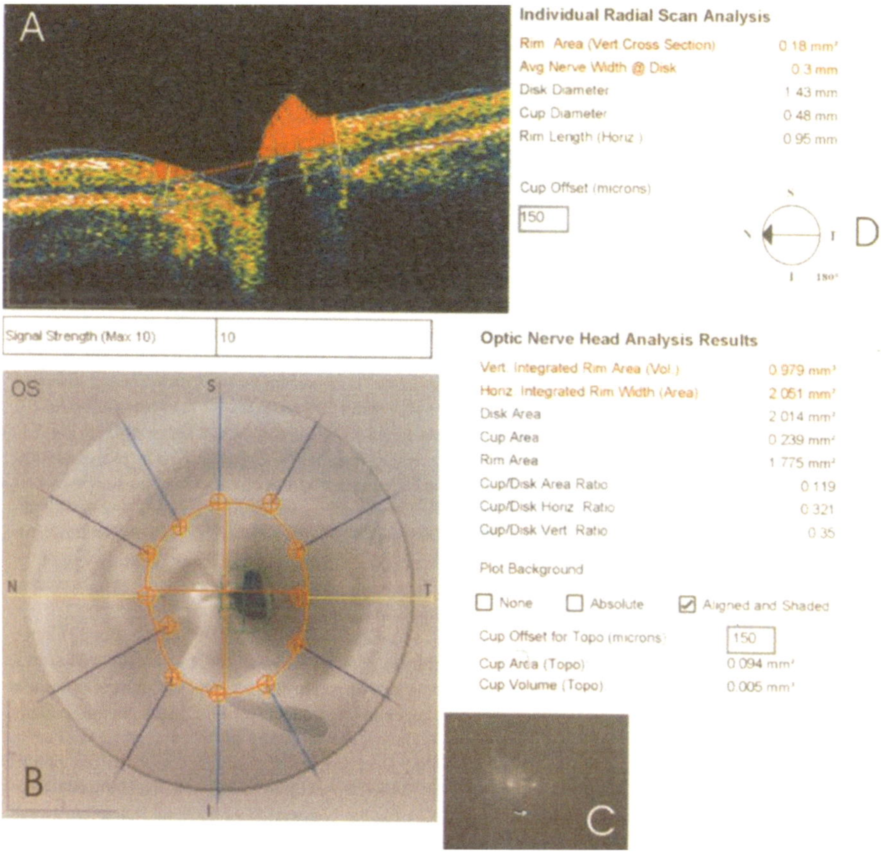

Figure 3.
Optic nerve head analysis report (adapted from Carl Zeiss OCT Manual).

lines consists of 128 A scans crossing an area of 4 mm in length vertically with a total scan time of 1.92 s. The optic nerve head analysis report consists of a B scan image of the optic nerve head taken horizontally and an overall gray scale image of the optic disc demonstrating the disc and the cup margins (**Figure 3**).

The parameters for individual radial scan analysis are derived from an algorithm which takes into account the location of the inner limiting membrane (ILM) and the termination of the retinal pigment epithelium (RPE layer)/Bruch's membrane. Since the RPE/Bruch's termination defines the edge of the disc margin the horizontal distance between the two points on the RPE/Bruch's termination gives the disc diameter. A second line is drawn 150 μm above and parallel to the one connecting the two points on the RPE/Bruch's termination. This is the plane that separates the rim from the cup. The cup diameter is the horizontal distance between the two points of intersection of this line with the ILM. Rim length is the difference between the cup diameter and the rim diameter. The rim area is total area above this line. The optic nerve head analysis is a conglomeration of all six radial scans arranged in a spoke pattern and interpolation of data between each of the scans created by smooth lines created around the disc and cup margins. Disc and cup areas are computed as the area within these margins, and rim area is calculated as the disc area minus cup area. The cup disc ratios (both horizontal and vertical) are calculated by the maximum distances of the disc and cup margins in the horizontal and vertical meridian, respectively. The vertical integrated rim area is an area interpolated around the discs of individual scans to define a rim volume. The horizontal integrated rim width is the mean of average nerve widths multiplied by the value of circumference of the disc. The major limitation of the fast scan is the need for interpolation of data between the spaces which assumes that the six scans each time has been centered exactly at the same line. Hence, significant eye movements during a scan lead to loss of focal defects.

8.1.2 The retinal nerve fiber layer (RNFL) analysis

The RNFL analysis involves a fast RNFL scan which takes approximately 1.9 s and acquires three fast circular scans 3.4 mm around the disc. This is time-efficient scan alignment and placement is required only once, each scan having an automated segmentation algorithm that detects the ILM boundary, the RNFL, and the ganglion cell body layer.

RNFL map comprises of six circular scans of 1.44, 1.69, 2.25, 2.73, and 3.40 mm radii. The scan size is 2.27 times the radius of the ONH. It helps to measure RNFL thickness with accuracy in various disc sizes. Centration of the circle around the disc is shown as an image adjacent to the scans and decentration of this circle can lead to erroneous results for RNFL thickness as closer circle position to the disc gives a thicker RNFL measurement while a position far away gives thinner readings.

The RNFL thickness is reported as overall average thickness and averages by quadrants and clock hours. The average RNFL thickness and various comparisons within the same and the other eye is also projected in a tabular form (**Figure 4**).

RNFL thickness map typically has a double hump pattern as the RNFL is thicker at the superior and inferior poles. The thickness of RNFL of a patient is compared to age matched normative data base and interpreted in different color codings. The green color encompasses the 5th to 95th percentile of the normative range for RNFL and is considered normal. The yellow color represents first to fifth percentile of the normal population and considered borderline. Anything below the first percentile

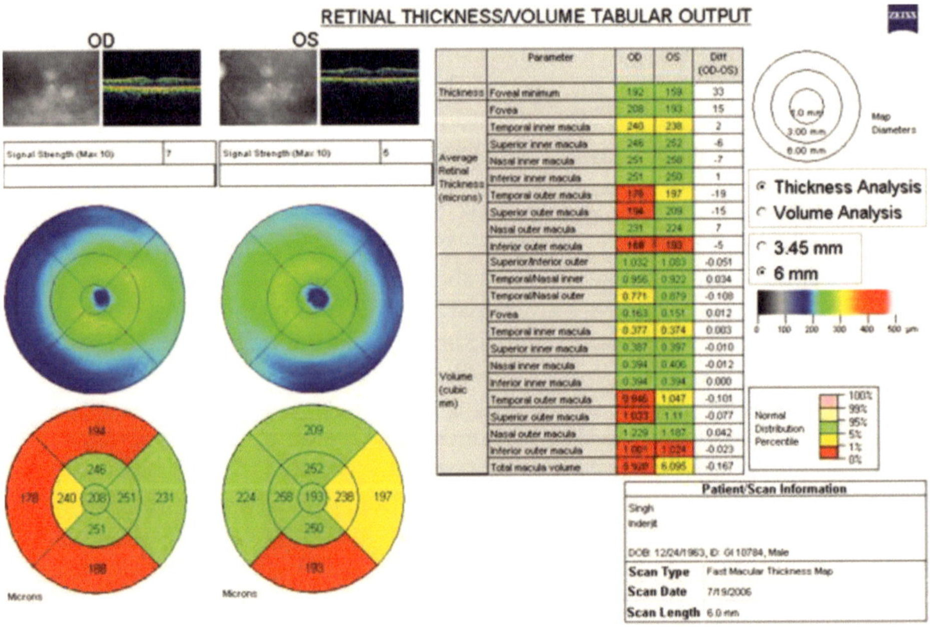

Figure 4.
Retinal nerve fiber layer thickness/volume tabular output.

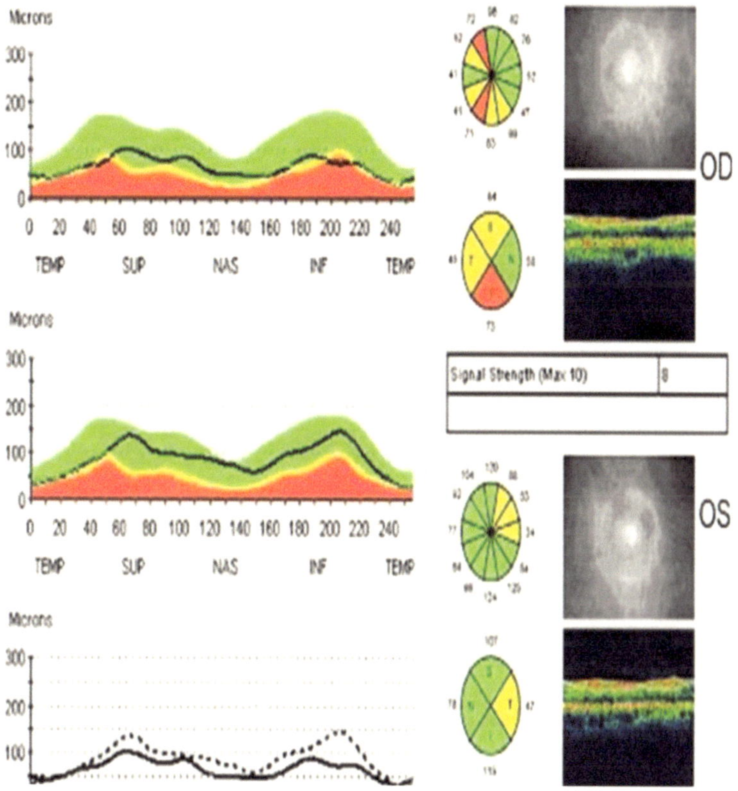

Figure 5.
RNFL thickness average analysis report (Stratus OCT: Carl Zeiss Meditec, Inc.).

is shown in red and considered outside normal limits. Values greater than 95th percentile are indicated in white and depicts above normal values (**Figure 5**).

8.2 Fourier domain OCT (FD-OCT) in glaucoma diagnosis

The newer generation Fourier-domain optical coherence tomography (FD-OCT) technology offers tremendous advances over the traditional time-domain (TD) technology in terms of speed and resolution. Currently, the Cirrus high-definition (HD)-OCT and RTVue 100 are commercially used to quantify peripapillary RNFL thickness in clinical practice. Studies indicate that RNFL thickness parameters measured on Cirrus OCT are reproducible and have high diagnostic sensitivity and specificity in discriminating between healthy and glaucomatous eyes [10, 11]. Furthermore, for the detection of glaucoma RNFL parameters of the RTVue-100 OCT have shown high specificity [12]. Studies indicate that ganglion cells located in the macular area are the earliest cells to be lost in glaucoma and hence this has led to utilize the less explored parameter of various OCT devices, the ganglion cell complex located in the macular region [13].

8.2.1 Optic nerve head scan pattern

The ONH scan is a combination of circular scans for RNFL thickness analysis and radial scans for ONH shape analysis. Combining circular scans and radial scans into one single pattern ensures that the RNFL scan and ONH scan naturally share same center. The scan time is only 0.5 s to help minimize any effect of eye movement. Hence the scan consists of 13 circles with diameters of 1.3–4.9 mm, which is used to create circumpapillary nerve fiber (NFL) map and 12 radial lines with 3.7 mm length, which are used to calculate the disc margin which forms the ONH scan. All B-scans (lines) are centered at the optic disc.

8.2.2 Three dimensional disc scan pattern

The three dimensional (3D) disc scan provides high definition OCT image both at horizontal and vertical direction for ONH. The 3D disc scan covers a default 5 mm × 5 mm square region and is adjustable. It contains 101 horizontal lines. The 3D disc scan contains a total of 51,813 A-scans and takes 2.2 s. The analysis includes B-scan fly through, 3D display, and en face summation of intensity in a retinal sub-layer or band. The 3D scan also creates a high definition OCT SLO projection as a baseline for registration of the ONH scan between multiple visits. Yellow indicates a borderline result. Thickness measures with a p-value less than 1% are colored red to indicate an outside normal limits result.

8.2.3 Diagnostic parameters

The RNFL thickness profile is divided into 16 sectors and the sector averages are displayed outside of RNFL thickness map. Thickness measurement is compared with normative database with a probability value (p-value) between 5 and 95% shown as green color to indicate within normal limits. Thickness measures with a p-value less than 5% are colored yellow to indicate a borderline result and a p-value less than 1% are colored red to indicate thickness outside normal limits (**Figure 6**).

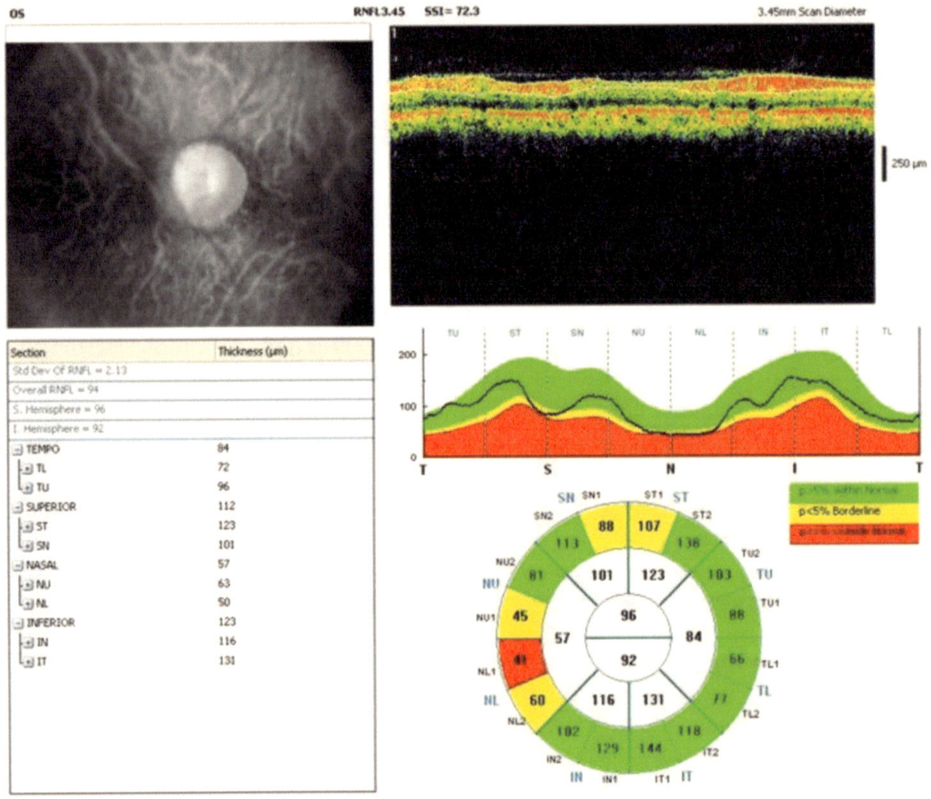

Figure 6.
RNFL thickness average analysis (Optovue A4 Version).

8.2.4 Ganglion cell complex

The diagnosis of glaucoma was improved by concentrating on the ganglion cell complex rather than the entire retinal thickness. The ganglion cell complex is a three layered structure consisting of the nerve fiber, ganglion cell and inner plexiform layers (**Figure 7**).

It has been shown that glaucoma predominantly causes thinning of the GCC [14, 15]. The GCC scan consists of three-dimensional scans of the macular region that samples the macula with 14,928 A-scans over a 7-mm square area. The scan pattern consists of 1 horizontal line and 15 vertical lines at 0.5-mm intervals. The center of the GCC scan is shifted 0.75 mm temporally to improve sampling of the temporal periphery.

The GCC scan quantifies the thickness in all three retina layers affected by glaucoma thereby causing the ganglion cell layer to become thinner as glaucoma progresses. Since the macula contains 50% of all ganglion cells in the retina, GCC scan analysis is a robust method of assessing early ganglion cell loss in glaucoma.

8.2.4.1 Ganglion cell map displays

Ganglion cell layer results are displayed in terms of three maps (**Figure 8**). The thickness map is color coded in a manner that brighter colors (red and orange) represent thicker areas and cooler colors (blue and green) represent thinner areas. Fovea has no ganglion cells and so is very thin (black spot).

In addition to the GCC thickness map, two other maps are also calculated and displayed on the analysis page for the GCC scan. A deviation map is calculated based on comparing the thickness map to the normative databases. The percent deviation is displayed with a color map where dark colors mean loss. Yellow and red are above average GCC (no loss). Blue is around 20% GCC loss and black is 50% loss or greater. The significance map is the GCC thickness map compared to the normal database at each single point, with probability values. Any point with thickness

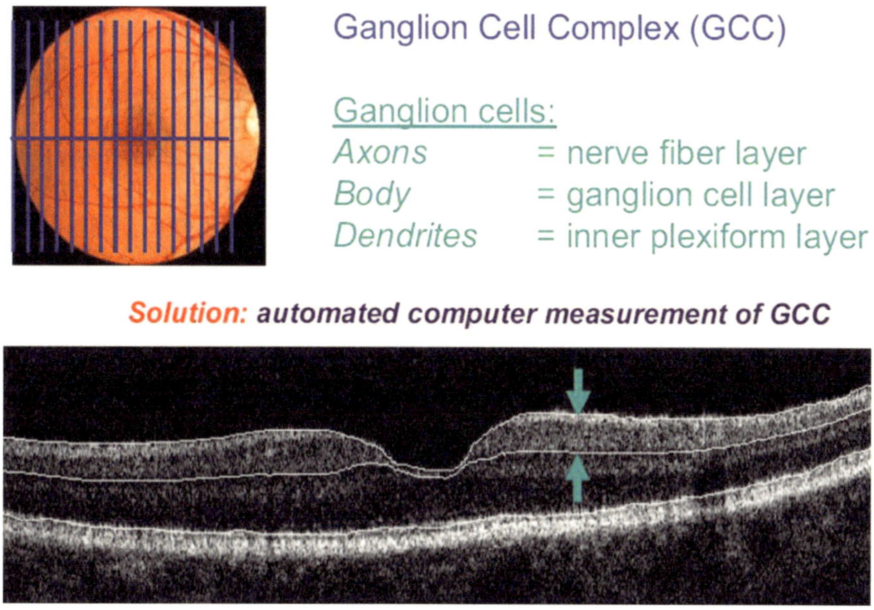

Figure 7.
Ganglion cell complex.

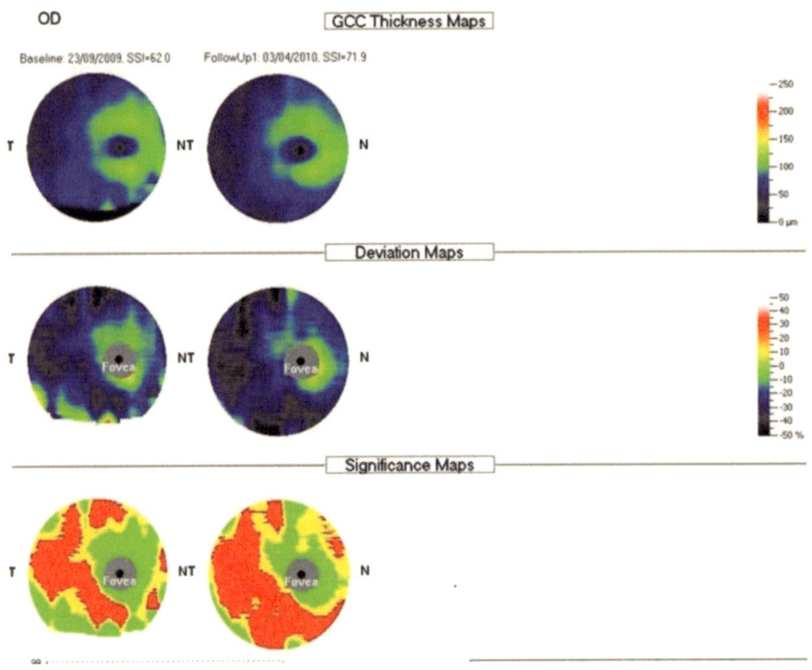

Figure 8.
GCC map displays (Optovue: RTVue Version A4).

under 5% of the normal population is labeled as borderline with a yellow color and thickness under 1% is labeled as outside normal limits and has a red color. A green color means above the 5% of normal population.

9. Determining progression using OCT

Glaucoma is a progressive disorder and monitoring progression forms a quintessential part of glaucoma management. Quantitative assessment of progression can be done in a predictable manner using OCT as compared to the qualitative and subjective assessment of the optic nerve head using optic disc photographs. There exists an inherent variability of each machine which is calculated in each machine by repeated measurements preferably the same day. Any change amounting to two to three times the standard deviation of the machine is taken as a real change in terms of progression. In Stratus OCT, the measurement variability is markedly lower for RNFL scans as compared to ONH analysis thereby making RNFL scans a better method in determining changes over time or what is termed as true progression.

Glaucoma progression is either event based or trend based according to statistical analysis. In event analysis, a threshold is determined and true progression is said to have occurred when a follow-up measurement exceeds this preestablished threshold. Any change below this threshold is considered to be due to natural age-related loss or measurement variability. Event analysis thus, is intended to identify a gradual change over time crossing the threshold or development of a sudden event that falls above the predetermined threshold. On the contrary, a trend analysis identifies progression by monitoring the behavior of a parameter over time. This method is therefore, less sensitive to sudden change and the variability among consecutive tests.

9.1 Progression with time domain OCT

Progression with time domain OCT mostly utilizes the RNFL thickness measurements as these have shown to discriminate well between normal and glaucomatous eyes [16, 17]. Both diffuse and localized glaucomatous RNFL defects in the peripapillary area have shown to have good reproducibility with low intra-test and inter-test variability and can be utilized in determining progression [18–24]. Based on the published data on the repeatability of mean RNFL thickness measurements, any decrease in thickness exceeding 6.4–8 μm can be considered to be abnormal and beyond the limits of test-retest variability with 95% tolerance [25]. These values are used only for mean peripapillary RNFL thickness and not for quadrants and clock hours as the variability is significantly higher in these areas owing to the shifts in scan locations.

The guided progression analysis (GPA) is a trend-based analysis that uses a linear regression to report change in overall mean RNFL thickness over time and also provides the significance of this change. The point of concern with the GPA analysis of Stratus OCT is that statistical significance reported doesn't take into consideration the rate of normal age-related loss. Therefore, some normal age-related changes may be reported as significant even though they do not represent true disease progression. The average age-related RNFL loss is expected to be between 0.16 and 0.31 μm/year [26–28].

9.2 Progression with spectral domain OCT

The substantial increase in SD-OCT scanning speed over TD-OCT makes scans less prone to eye movement artifacts. Studies have reported excellent intra-visit and inter-visit measurement reproducibility for SD-OCT [29–34], superior to TD-OCT [35–37]. This makes the SD-OCT a potential tool in monitoring glaucoma progression.

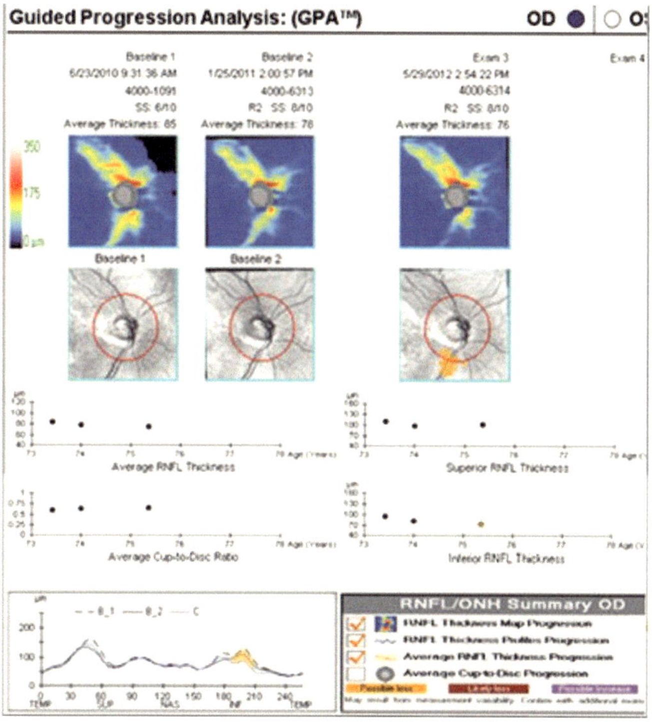

Figure 9.
Cirrus SD-OCT RNFL-guided progression analysis (adapted Carl Zeiss Meditec, Dublin, CA).

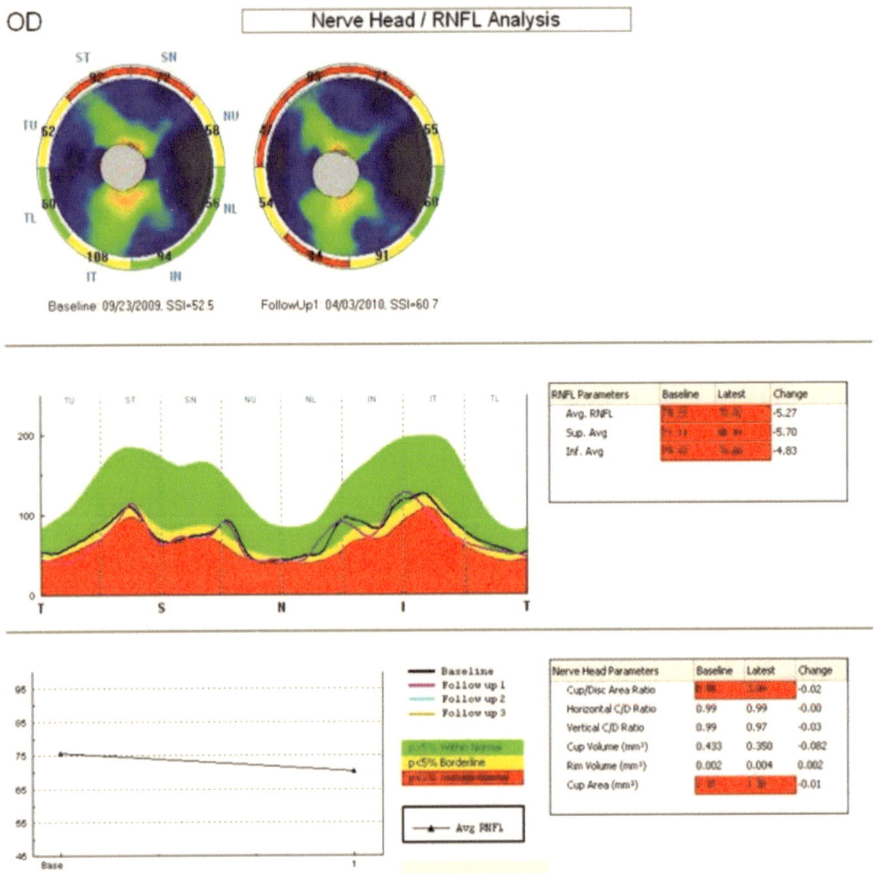

Figure 10.
RNFL change analysis (adapted: Optovue, Fremont, CA).

Ganglion cell complex diagnostic accuracy for detecting glaucoma has been shown to be similar to that of peripapillary RNFL thickness making it potentially valuable for monitoring glaucoma progression [38–42].

Progression analysis is currently available with Cirrus HD-OCT (Carl Zeiss Meditec, Dublin, CA) and RTVue (Optovue, Fremont, CA). Of these two devices, statistical analyses in form of event- and trend-based mechanism for progression detection is available only in the Cirrus HD-OCT. Data sampling of the RNFL is obtained from the 3.4-mm diameter peripapillary circle and the software also displays RNFL thickness changes from baseline for each pixel in the scanned area. Possible or likely RNFL thickness loss is reported if change exceeds the expected test-retest variability in a single or two consecutive follow-up examinations, respectively. In addition, linear regression is performed to determine the rate of change, confidence limits, and statistical significance of the trend (**Figure 9**).

The RTVue offers progression analysis that includes side-by-side RNFL thickness measurements and overlay of the RNFL profiles for the consecutive scans. The RT Vue also provides similar analysis for ganglion cell complex thickness along with thickness change plots (**Figure 10**). However, a formal statistical analysis of change over time is not currently included in the latest version of the software for this device (version 6.1) (**Figure 11**).

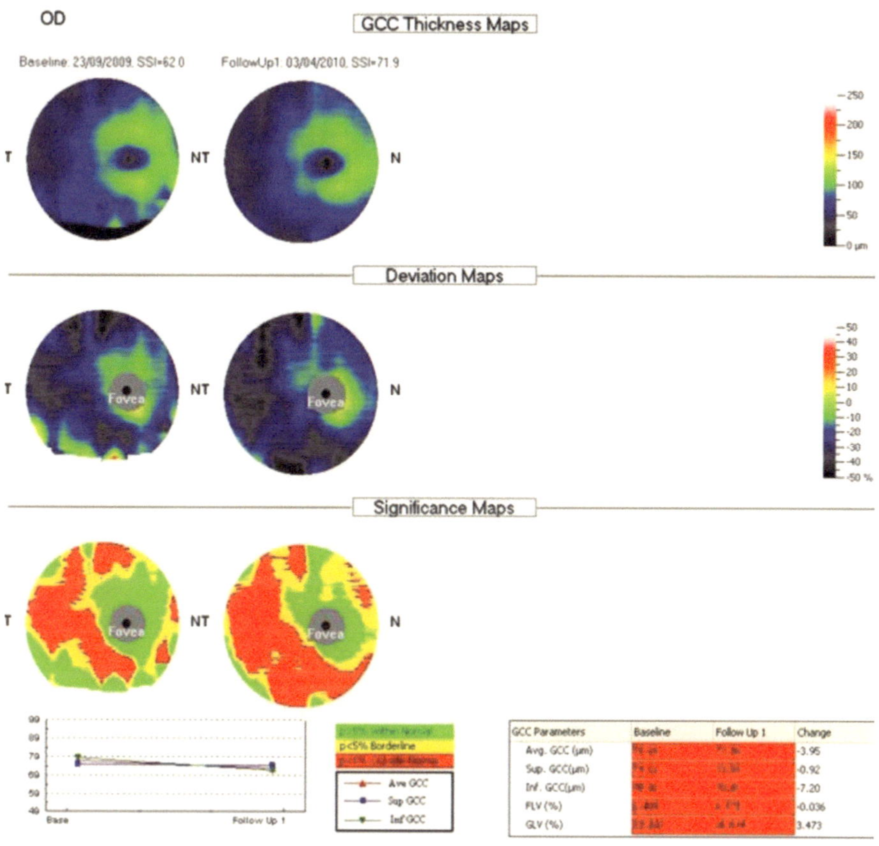

Figure 11.
Ganglion cell analysis showing progression (adapted: Optovue, Fremont, CA).

10. Anterior segment OCT (AS-OCT)

Anterior segment OCT (AS-OCT) imaging initially described by Izatt et al. using the same wavelength of light as retinal OCT [43]. However, the 830 nm wavelength was found to be suboptimal for imaging the angle due to limited penetration through scattering tissue such as the sclera. Hence, a newer OCT imaging of the anterior segment with a longer wavelength of 1310 nm was developed that had the advantages of better penetration through sclera [44]. Currently, there are two dedicated anterior segment devices commercially available. The SL-OCT (Heidelberg Engineering) and the Visante (Carl Zeiss Meditec, Inc.) Newer Fourier domain anterior segment OCT devices however have been developed, and these allow rapid three-dimensional cube scanning of the anterior segment.

10.1 Qualitative assessment using AS-OCT

An important landmark to identify when interpreting AS-OCT images is the scleral spur. This is visible as an inward projection of the sclera at the junction between the inner scleral and corneal curvatures. Studies have shown that scleral spur may not be visible in 25% cases [45]. The apposition between the iris and the inner corneo-scleral wall has been used in several studies as a qualitative method of detecting closure of the anterior chamber angle [46, 47]. The degree of apposition however may not correlate exactly with appositional closure as defined by gonioscopy.

10.2 Quantitative assessment using AS-OCT

An in-built software in most of the AS-OCT helps in quantitative measurement of the anterior chamber angle. Several parameters designated for the quantitative analysis has shown good reproducibility [48–50]. Difficulty in visualizing the scleral spur and the wide natural variation in angle anatomy within the same eye as well as between eyes are limiting factors in the routine use of quantitative measurement for angle assessment.

The various quantitative parameters reported are as follows (**Figure 12a–c**):

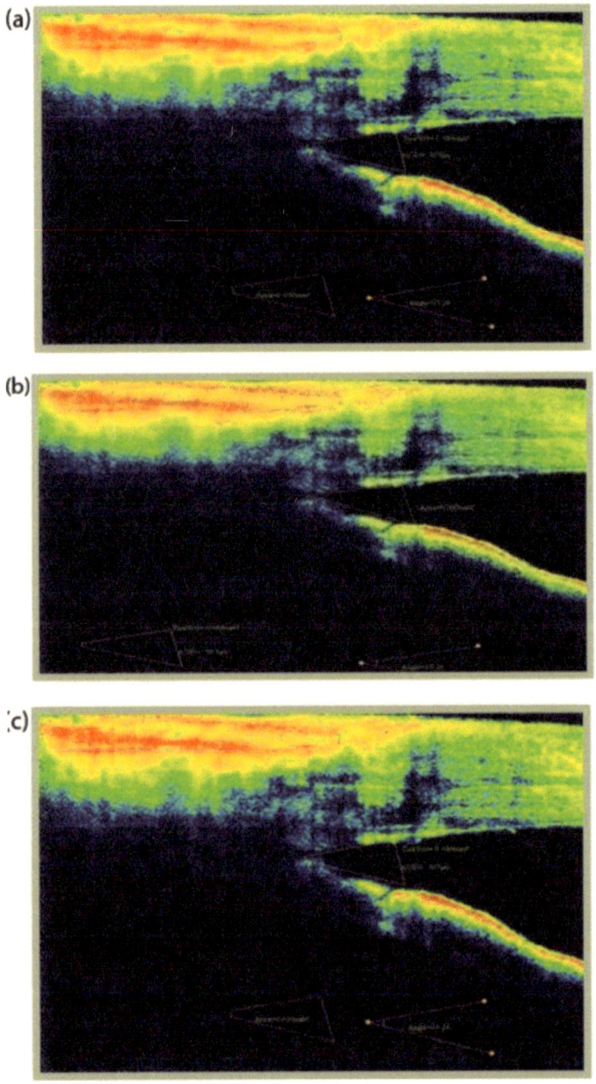

Figure 12.
Quantitative measurement of (a) angle opening distance using RTVue anterior segment OCT, (b) angle recess area using RTVue anterior segment OCT, and (c) trabeculo-iris space area using RTVue anterior segment OCT.

a. Angle opening distance (AOD in mm): it is the perpendicular distance between a point 500 μm (AOD 500) or 750 μm (AOD750) anterior to the scleral spur and the opposing iris.

b. Angle recess area (ARA in mm^2): it is a triangular area (ARA 500 or 750) bounded by the AOD 500 or 750, the anterior iris surface, and the inner corneo-scleral wall.

Trabecular space area (TISA in mm^2): it is the trapezoidal area (TISA 500 or 750) bounded by the AOD 500 or 750, the anterior iris surface, the inner corneo-scleral wall, and the perpendicular distance between the scleral spur and the opposing iris.

10.3 Clinical applications

In clinical glaucoma practice, AS-OCT is used as an adjunct to gonioscopy. It can act as a substitute when gonioscopy is not feasible due to corneal pathology or lack of patient co-operation. Furthermore, it is extremely useful as a patient education tool, to explain the pathophysiology of angle closure to patients before any laser procedures like peripheral iridotomy. Its advantages over gonioscopy lie in the fact that it is a non-contact procedure and can be performed under dark conditions allowing angle assessment during physiological mydriasis. A major limitation however is its inability to visualize the structures behind the iris. This limits its ability in diagnosing the posterior mechanisms of angle closure such as iridociliary lesions and plateau iris. AS-OCT may also be used to visualize trabeculectomy blebs and anterior segment implants such as drainage devices and keratoprosthesis—however, the clinical value in these situations appears to be limited.

11. Conclusion

Advances in OCT technology have made it possible to apply OCT in a wide variety of applications. The high depth and transversal resolution in OCT and the ability to decouple depth resolution from transverse resolution make it an important tool in ophthalmic imaging. Few other advantages are high probing depth in scattering media, contact free, and non-invasive operation, and the possibility to create various function-dependent image contrasting methods.

11.1 Limitations

1. Because OCT utilizes light waves (unlike ultrasound which uses sound waves), media opacities such as vitreous hemorrhage, dense cataract, or corneal opacities can interfere with optimal imaging.

2. Motion artifacts: eye movements can sometimes diminish the quality of the image. However with the spectral domain shortened acquisition, time often results in fewer motion related artifacts.

3. Learning curve: acquiring good quality images are an art and has a learning curve. Although with the advent of newer technologies, such as spectral domain acquisition or the use of eye tracking equipment, the likelihood of such acquisition error has been reduced dramatically.

Author details

Baswati Sahoo[1*] and Julie Pegu[2]

1 Ahalia Hospital, Abu Dhabi, United Arab Emirates

2 Dr. Shroffs Charity Eye hospital, New Delhi, India

*Address all correspondence to: bpsceh@gmail.com

References

[1] Bathija R, Gupta N, Zangwill L, et al. Changing definition of glaucoma. Journal of Glaucoma. 1998;7(3):165-169

[2] Gordon MO, Torri V, Miglior S. Validated prediction model for the development of primary open-angle glaucoma in individuals with ocular hypertension. Ophthalmology. 2007;**114**:10-19

[3] Sommer A, Katz J, Quigley HA, Miller NR, Robin AL, Richter RC. Clinically detectable nerve fiber atrophy precedes the onset of glaucomatous field loss. Archives of Ophthalmology. 1991;**109**:77-83

[4] Medeiros FA, Zangwill LM, Bowd C, Sample PA, Weinreb RN. Use of progressive glaucomatous optic disk change as the reference standard for evaluation of diagnostic tests in glaucoma. American Journal of Ophthalmology. 2005;**139**:1010-1018

[5] Caprioli J, Nouri-Mahdavi K, Law SK, Badalà F. Optic disc imaging in perimetrically normal eyes of glaucoma patients with unilateral field loss. Transactions of the American Ophthalmological Society. 2006;**104**:202-211

[6] Airaksinen PJ, Tuulonen A, Werner EB. Clinical evaluation of the optic disc and retinal nerve fiber layer. In: Ritch R, Shields MB, Krupin T, editors. The Glaucomas. St. Louis: Mosby; 1996. pp. 617-657

[7] Sull AC, Vuong LN, Price LL, et al. Comparison of spectral/Fourier domain optical coherence tomography instruments for assessment of normal macular thickness. Retina. 2010;**30**:235-245

[8] de Boer JF, Cense B, Park BH, et al. Improved signal-to-noise ratio in spectral-domain compared with time-domain optical coherence tomography. Optics Letters. 2003;**28**:2067-2069

[9] Leitgeb R, Hitzenberger C, Fercher A. Performance of Fourier domain vs. time domain optical coherence tomography. Optics Express. 2003;**11**:889-894

[10] Mwanza JC, Oakley JD, Budenz DL, Anderson DR. Cirrus Optical Coherence Tomography Normative Database Study Group. Ability of cirrus HD-OCT optic nerve head parameters to discriminate normal from glaucomatous eyes. Ophthalmology. 2011;**118**:241-280

[11] Sung KR, Na JH, Lee Y. Glaucoma diagnostic capabilities of optic nerve head parameters as determined by cirrus HD optical coherence tomography. Journal of Glaucoma. 2012;**21**:498-504

[12] Paul C. To assess the glaucoma diagnostic ability of Fourier domain optical coherence tomography. American Journal of Engineering Research. 2013;**10**:155-169

[13] Hood DC, Raza AS, de Moraes CG, Liebmann JM, Ritch R. Glaucomatous damage of the macula. Progress in Retinal and Eye Research. 2013;**32**:1-21

[14] Medeiros FA, Zangwill LM, Bowd C, Vessani RM, Susanna R Jr, Weinreb RN. Evaluation of retinal nerve fiber layer, optic nerve head, and macular thickness measurements for glaucoma detection using optical coherence tomography. American Journal of Ophthalmology. 2005;**139**:44-55

[15] Budenz DL, Michael A, Chang RT, McSoley J, Katz J. Sensitivity and specificity of the StratusOCT for perimetric glaucoma. Ophthalmology. 2005;**112**:3-9

[16] Medeiros FA, Zangwill LM, Bowd C, Weinreb RN. Comparison of the GDx VCC scanning laser polarimeter, HRT II confocal scanning laser ophthalmoscope, and stratus OCT optical coherence tomograph for the detection of glaucoma. Archives of Ophthalmology. 2004;**122**:827-837

[17] Wollstein G, Ishikawa H, Wang J, Beaton SA, Schuman JS. Comparison of three optical coherence tomography scanning areas for detection of glaucomatous damage. American Journal of Ophthalmology. 2005;**139**:39-43

[18] Bowd C, Zangwill LM, Berry CC, et al. Detecting early glaucoma by assessment of retinal nerve fiber layer thickness and visual function. Investigative Ophthalmology & Visual Science. 2001;**42**:1993-2003

[19] Blumenthal EZ, Williams JM, Weinreb RN, Girkin CA, Berry CC, Zangwill LM. Reproducibility of nerve fiber layer thickness measurements by use of optical coherence tomography. Ophthalmology. 2000;**107**:2278-2282

[20] Budenz DL, Chang RT, Huang X, Knighton RW, Tielsch JM. Reproducibility of retinal nerve fiber thickness measurements using the stratus OCT in normal and glaucomatous eyes. Investigative Ophthalmology & Visual Science. 2005;**46**:2440-2443

[21] Budenz DL, Fredette MJ, Feuer WJ, Anderson DR. Reproducibility of peripapillary retinal nerve fiber thickness measurements with stratus OCT in glaucomatous eyes. Ophthalmology. 2008;**115**:661-666

[22] Paunescu LA, Schuman JS, Price LL, et al. Reproducibility of nerve fiber thickness, macular thickness, and optic nerve head measurements using Stratus OCT. Investigative Ophthalmology & Visual Science. 2004;**45**:1716-1724

[23] Schuman JS, Pedut-Kloizman T, Hertzmark E, et al. Reproducibility of nerve fiber layer thickness measurements using optical coherence tomography. Ophthalmology. 1996;**103**:1889-1898

[24] Gurses-Ozden R, Teng C, Vessani R, Zafar S, Liebmann JM, Ritch R. Macular and retinal nerve fiber layer thickness measurement reproducibility using optical coherence tomography (OCT-3). Journal of Glaucoma. 2004;**13**:238-244

[25] Lee EJ, Kim TW, Park KH, Seong M, Kim H, Kim DM. Ability of stratus OCT to detect progressive retinal nerve fiber layer atrophy in glaucoma. Investigative Ophthalmology & Visual Science. 2009;**50**:662-668

[26] Budenz DL, Anderson DR, Varma R, et al. Determinants of normal retinal nerve fiber layer thickness measured by stratus OCT. Ophthalmology. 2007;**114**:1046-1052

[27] Parikh RS, Parikh SR, Sekhar GC, Prabakaran S, Babu JG, Thomas R. Normal age-related decay of retinal nerve fiber layer thickness. Ophthalmology. 2007;**114**:921-926

[28] Harwerth RS, Wheat JL, Rangaswamy NV. Age-related losses of retinal ganglion cells and axons. Investigative Ophthalmology & Visual Science. 2008;**49**:4437-4443

[29] Garas A, Vargha P, Hollo G. Reproducibility of retinal nerve fiber layer and macular thickness measurement with the RTVue-100 optical coherence tomograph. Ophthalmology. 2010;**117**:738-746

[30] Gonzalez-Garcia AO, Vizzeri G, Bowd C, Medeiros FA, Zangwill LM, Weinreb RN. Reproducibility of RTVue retinal nerve fiber layer

thickness and optic disc measurements and agreement with stratus optical coherence tomography measurements. American Journal of Ophthalmology. 2009;**147**:1067-1074

[31] Lee SH, Kim SH, Kim TW, Park KH, Kim DM. Reproducibility of retinal nerve fiber thickness measurements using the test-retest function of spectral OCT/SLO in normal and glaucomatous eyes. Journal of Glaucoma. 2010;**19**:637-642

[32] Li JP, Wang XZ, Fu J, Li SN, Wang NL. Reproducibility of RTVue retinal nerve fiber layer thickness and optic nerve head measurements in normal and glaucoma eyes. Chinese Medical Journal. 2010;**123**:1898-1903

[33] Mwanza JC, Chang RT, Budenz DL, et al. Reproducibility of peripapillary retinal nerve fiber layer thickness and optic nerve head parameters measured with CirrusTM HD-OCT in glaucomatous eyes. Investigative Ophthalmology & Visual Science. 2010;**51**:5724-5730

[34] Menke MN, Knecht P, Sturm V, Dabov S, Funk J. Reproducibility of nerve fiber layer thickness measurements using 3D fourier-domain OCT. Investigative Ophthalmology & Visual Science. 2008;**49**:5386-5391

[35] Schuman JS. Spectral domain optical coherence tomography for glaucoma (an AOS thesis). Transactions of the American Ophthalmological Society. 2008;**106**:426-458

[36] Leung CK, Cheung CY, Weinreb RN, et al. Retinal nerve fiber layer imaging with spectral-domain optical coherence tomography: A variability and diagnostic performance study. Ophthalmology. 2009;**116**:1257-1263

[37] Kim JS, Ishikawa H, Sung KR, et al. Retinal nerve fibre layer thickness measurement reproducibility improved with spectral domain optical coherence tomography. The British Journal of Ophthalmology. 2009;**93**:1057-1063

[38] Garas A, Vargha P, Hollo G. Diagnostic accuracy of nerve fibre layer, macular thickness and optic disc measurements made with the RTVue-100 optical coherence tomograph to detect glaucoma. Eye. 2011;**25**:57-65

[39] Kim NR, Lee ES, Seong GJ, et al. Comparing the ganglion cell complex and retinal nerve fibre layer measurements by Fourier domain OCT to detect glaucoma in high myopia. The British Journal of Ophthalmology. [published online ahead of print October 17, 2010]

[40] Rao HL, Zangwill LM, Weinreb RN, Sample PA, Alencar LM, Medeiros FA. Comparison of different spectral domain optical coherence tomography scanning areas for glaucoma diagnosis. Ophthalmology. 2010;**117**:1692-1699

[41] Tan O, Chopra V, Lu AT, et al. Detection of macular ganglion cell loss in glaucoma by Fourier-domain optical coherence tomography. Ophthalmology. 2009;**116**:2305-2314

[42] Tan O, Li G, Lu AT, Varma R, Huang D. Mapping of macular substructures with optical coherence tomography for glaucoma diagnosis. Ophthalmology. 2008;**115**:949-956

[43] Izatt JA, Hee MR, Swanson EA, et al. Micrometer-scale resolution imaging of the anterior eye in vivo with optical coherence tomography. Archives of Ophthalmology. 1994;**112**:1584-1589

[44] Radhakrishnan S, Rollins AM, Roth JE, et al. Real-time optical coherence tomography of the anterior segment at 1310 nm. Archives of Ophthalmology. 2001;**119**:1179-1185

[45] Sakata LM, Lavanya R, Friedman DS, et al. Assessment of the scleral spur

in anterior segment optical coherence tomography images. Archives of Ophthalmology. 2008;**126**:181-185

[46] Nolan WP, See JL, Chew PT, et al. Detection of primary angle closure using anterior segment OCT in Asian eyes. Ophthalmology. 2007;**114**:33-39

[47] Lavanya R, Foster PJ, Sakata LM, et al. Screening for narrow angles in the Singapore population: Evaluation of new non-contact screening methods. Ophthalmology. 2008;**115**:1720-1727

[48] Radhakrishnan S, Goldsmith J, Westphal V, et al. Comparison of coherence tomography and ultrasound biomicroscopy for detection of narrow anterior chamber angles. Archives of Ophthalmology. 2005;**128**:1053-1059

[49] Fukuda S, Kawana K, Yasuno Y, et al. Repeatability and reproducibility of anterior ocular biometric measurements with 2-D and 3-D optical coherence tomography. Journal of Cataract and Refractive Surgery. 2010;**36**:1867-1873

[50] Tan AN, Sauren LD, de Brabander J, et al. Reproducibility of anterior chamber angle measurements with anterior segment OCT. Investigative Ophthalmology & Visual Science. 2011;**52**:2095-2099